THE GIFT OF
ADVERSITY

JEREMY P. TARCHER/PENGUIN
a member of Penguin Group (USA)
New York

NORMAN E. ROSENTHAL, M.D.

THE GIFT OF
ADVERSITY

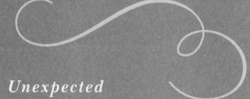

The Unexpected

Benefits of

Life's Difficulties,

Setbacks, and

Imperfections

JEREMY P. TARCHER/PENGUIN
Published by the Penguin Group
Penguin Group (USA) LLC
375 Hudson Street
New York, New York 10014

USA • Canada • UK • Ireland • Australia
New Zealand • India • South Africa • China

penguin.com
A Penguin Random House Company

First trade paperback edition 2014
Copyright © 2013 by Norman E. Rosenthal, M.D.

The writing exercise on page 325 is from *Opening Up: The Healing Power of
Expressing Emotions* by James W. Pennebaker, Ph.D., 1997, the Guildford Press.
Reprinted by permission of the Guildford Press.

"One Art" on page 177 is from *The Complete Poems 1927–1979* by Elizabeth Bishop.
Copyright © 1979, 1983 by Alice Helen Methfessel. Reprinted by permission
of Farrar, Straus and Giroux LLC.

Most Tarcher/Penguin books are available at special quantity discounts for bulk purchase for sales promotions,
premiums, fund-raising, and educational needs. Special books or book excerpts also can be created to fit specific
needs. For details, write: Special.Markets@us.penguingroup.com.

The Library of Congress has catalogued the hardcover edition as follows:

Rosenthal, Norman E.
  The gift of adversity: the unexpected benefits of life's
difficulties, setbacks, and imperfections / Norman E. Rosenthal, M.D.
  p.   cm.
  Includes index.
  ISBN 978-0-399-16371-5
  1. Disappointment.   2. Adjustment (Psychology).   3. Adaptability (Psychology).
4. Resilience (Personality trait).   5. Rosenthal, Norman E.   I. Title.
  BF575.D57R67   2013   2013015299
  155.2'4—dc23

ISBN 978-0-399-16885-7 (paperback)

Printed in the United States of America
10 9 8 7 6 5 4 3 2 1

Book design by Ellen Cipriano

FOR

NORMAN ROSENTHAL

(1920–1942)

AND ARI

CONTENTS

PART II. ADULTHOOD

PART III. HEROES

PART IV. FAREWELLS

INTRODUCTION

Sweet are the uses of adversity,
Which, like the toad, ugly and venomous,
Wears yet a precious jewel in his head.

—SHAKESPEARE, *AS YOU LIKE IT*

That which does not kill us makes us stronger.

—FRIEDRICH NIETZSCHE

He who learns must suffer. And even in our sleep, pain
that cannot forget falls drop by drop upon the heart,
and in our own despair, against our will, comes wisdom
to us by the awful grace of God.

—AESCHYLUS, *AGAMEMNON*

One way to think about this book is as a collection of stories that
happen to be true. They are stories I have collected through life's
journey, stories I have told to myself and others that cluster around a
theme: What has life dealt me and what have I learned from it? What

wisdom have I gleaned from the fascinating people whom fortune has put in my path and the curious times in which I have lived?

Somehow it is part of my nature, whenever something curious or unexpected happens, to ask myself, "What can I learn from this?" As I reflected on the stories I have collected, I reached an unexpected conclusion: All of them dealt with some sort of adversity, plus what I had learned from it. It has been said that you cannot become a master sailor on calm seas; so too you cannot navigate life successfully without learning how to handle adversity. To be sure, adversity is by its very nature painful and unwelcome. The trick then is how to move beyond these initial feelings and find something of value in the experience. That is the essence of this book: Put simply, the lessons embedded in these stories are the sweet uses of adversity. What does not kill us, to paraphrase Nietzsche, makes us stronger—but only if we learn from our mistakes and misfortunes.

It makes sense from an evolutionary point of view that we have the innate tools for such learning. Those ancient ones who learned best from danger, obstacles, setbacks, and reversals of fortune were more likely to survive long enough to transmit their DNA to future generations. Even so, although our ability to learn from adversity may be a highly selected trait, it can no doubt be greatly improved by experience and guidance, as I hope this book will show.

Adversity, it seems to me, can be divided into three categories. First, there is the adversity that results from plain bad luck—such as being in the wrong place at the wrong time, or being born with some genetic disease. Second is the adversity that we bring upon ourselves by making some mistake or error of judgment. The pain of this type of adversity is compounded by feelings of guilt and shame at having been responsible for the misfortune. Finally, there is the adversity that we actually seek out, as when we take a calculated risk, set off on an adventure, or let slip the dogs of war. Although adversity is not generally the stated goal of such an enterprise, it is an accepted and integral part of the process. Each type of adversity carries its own challenges and has the potential to yield its own form of wisdom. All will be represented in one form or another in this book.

As a psychiatrist, whenever things go wrong in the lives of my patients, I am always inclined to ask them: "Has anything like this ever happened to you before? What did you do then? And how did it work out?" Then, after the issue is sufficiently resolved, I often ask, "What lesson can you take from this event? How can you do things differently to prevent it from happening in the future?" It is natural for me to ask these questions, not only as a result of my training, but because they are the same questions I always ask myself—and have done as long as I can remember—whenever things don't work out as I had hoped. Over time these lessons accumulate, and, if we are lucky, in the words of Aeschylus, drop by drop comes wisdom, the bittersweet fruit of adversity. Crises are learning opportunities. If we can begin to draw connections between what we have learned from crises, we can work out a systematic way of dealing with them. Research shows that many people become happier as they get older. Perhaps that is a result of the wisdom we acquire over the years, which helps us avoid trouble when possible and deal better with it when it arises.

In my work with patients and in my writings, I often use stories to illustrate points, because I have always loved stories and gained a lot from them. Perhaps we are wired to learn from stories, since that is how experience has been recorded and communicated since the beginning of human time. Stories speak to both the heart and the mind: If they fail to move us, we are likely to learn less from them. So I have chosen stories as my main medium for communicating whatever wisdom you may find in these pages. Where appropriate, I buttress my stories with relevant research. I also conclude, in the spirit of Aesop, with a take-home message or two to summarize the point of each story. It is my hope that these takeaways will be a tool to help you remember and use the lessons that I and others took away from these events.

Although some of the stories in this book come from my own experiences, in many instances I am only the narrator, relating events that occurred in the lives of some of the intriguing people I have encountered: family members, friends, patients, and colleagues, as well as people I have had the good fortune to meet, or who have taken part in my research studies and writing projects. Through these experiences, I have had a privileged window into many different worlds.

A few disclaimers: Some of the adversity I will describe took place on a horrendous scale, such as what occurred in Nazi Germany or apartheid South Africa, in which I grew up, and many people suffered horribly as a result of both these fascist regimes. You will meet in this book people who have experienced adversity at that level: for example, the servants who helped to raise me and Holocaust survivors, including the great author and neurologist Viktor Frankl, whom I was fortunate enough to meet during the last years of his life. You will also meet people who have suffered homelessness, or the torment of severe mental illness and drug abuse. In all these cases, I do not wish to compare their profound suffering with anything I have experienced myself. My life has been for the most part a lucky one.

So this book is not intended to belong to the genre designed to draw attention to specific horrors endured by the author. Nor is it intended to be encyclopedic with regard to all possible adversities that a person might ever encounter. Instead, my goals in this book are twofold: first, to share some of the setbacks, reversals, and imperfections I and others have experienced, along with the unexpected insights they have provided; and second, to suggest ways in which you might benefit from these insights too.

Some chapters are devoted to methods for overcoming adversity, such as meditation, developing healthy habits, and—no surprise here—talking about traumatic experiences or writing about them—in other words, turning experiences into stories.

In summary, I hope you will find the stories in this book interesting in their own right, and that they will stimulate you to think about the adversity you have experienced, what you have learned from it, and how you can use that wisdom going forward. The take-home message of this book is that even when life is at its most painful and difficult, it has meaning and value. Even when things are really awful, some good can come of them. Our times of struggle yield gifts and riches that are worth harvesting, because they continue to nourish us throughout life's journey.

PART I

YOUTH

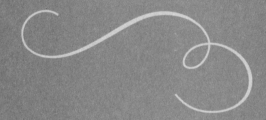

Chapter 1

The Thumbs Must Go

If a thing's worth doing, it's worth doing well.
—PROVERB

If a thing is worth doing, it is worth doing badly.
—G. K. CHESTERTON

My first-grade classroom was a prefabricated hut, made out of what seemed to me like reinforced cardboard, set on a concrete slab. What I recall most about it is the smell of leather from the backpacks in which we hauled our rudimentary items to and from school. Besides holding up the roof, cardboard played a role in the lessons too.

I remember one particular art project vividly, because it was a turning point for me. In this assignment, we were each given a large sheet of white cardboard on which various parts of a clown's body were outlined. Our task was to color in the clown's body parts with crayons, then cut them out and join the head, arms, and legs to the body using brass-plated fasteners. Then you could move the limbs up and down to make the clown do jumping jacks.

I started the project, but soon realized it was not going well. In retrospect, my fine motor control left a lot to be desired. Of course, nobody tested kids for fine motor control in those days, but I didn't need any test. I got the picture by simply glancing at the boy beside me. There I was laboring down the inner aspect of one arm toward the hand, while he was all the way around the hand of *his* clown, and barreling past the elbow. I looked back down at my clown's hand, still trapped in its cardboard moorings, and realized that if I tried to get it exactly right, my clown might not get done at all.

That was unacceptable! But how could I get it done? The fingers looked manageable, because they were all bunched together, but the thumb stuck out—as thumbs do—long, spindly, and difficult. And in that moment, I realized what I had to do: *The thumb must go!* And with that insight, I snipped it off.

From then on, all went smoothly. When I got to the bottom of the second arm, the course of action was clear. Again: *The thumb must go!* And in one snip, the second thumb was gone. By the end of the hour, the body parts were all cut out and I had managed to articulate the joints. My clown could do jumping jacks along with everyone else's, and he looked okay to me. So when we were all encouraged to come up to the table and show the teacher our work, I did so.

The teacher's attention was divided among many students, so she didn't have much time for individual comments—and the clowns all looked pretty much the same. But her eye did pause on mine for a moment and she said, "That clown's got no thumbs," before drifting on to her next observation.

The most important part of the lesson, as far as I was concerned, was that amputating the clown's thumbs had no significant consequences. I got the job done in time. I had a working clown. And apart from the teacher's one offhand remark, I can't recall anyone saying anything about the matter of the thumbs.

Many times since then, when I encounter some minor obstacle that's holding up an important task, I say to myself, "The thumbs must go!" And there and then, I know what to do.

On a recent visit to Israel, I was chatting with a cousin who is a lawyer for Israel's thriving technology industry. In fact, he told me that Israel ranks third in the world after Silicon Valley and the greater Boston area as a technology hub. How was it, I asked him, that such a small country could achieve such technological success? There had to be many factors at play, he said, then added, "Somehow they always seem to figure out shortcuts. As they say, 'The great is the enemy of the good.' Why wait for a product to be perfect before putting it on the market? Put out a beta version and let the marketplace work out the bugs." I smiled to myself. That's what my clown was, I realized—a beta version.

I HAVE SOMETIMES thought about how the lesson of the clown has influenced me throughout my life. His thumbs must have been part of my thinking when I embarked upon the most important experiment of my research career. The study in question involved exposing nine people with seasonal affective disorder (SAD) to two different types of lighting—bright white light and dim yellow light. The experiment was the first controlled study of light therapy for SAD, and the first to show bright light to be an effective treatment for the condition. The paper became a citation classic and opened up a whole new field of research.

In the beginning, however, because of our limited budget, we had to adopt certain shortcuts. For example, we had to improvise the dim light condition. We could think of no better way to dim the light than to attach brown paper inside the plastic screen of the light box. The overall effect was inartful—to say the least. Yet so powerful was the effect of bright light for SAD that it overcame all the shortcomings of the study. That research was replicated many times over and has been helping people all over the world for more than thirty years, so I'm certainly glad that I took a chance with a beta version.

I had a very different experience many years later, when I opened a private business to test out new drugs for psychiatric disorders, such as depression and anxiety. Exquisite attention was paid to every aspect of each study's design and implementation. No thumbs were cut. On the contrary, every fingernail was carefully clipped and buffed. And what resulted from all this meticulous attention to detail? Not much. A few studies (of the dozens we conducted) yielded results that were of some value in clinical practice, but overall, the drugs we tested were similar to others already in use. Therefore the results, even when significant and positive, usually made little difference.

As the proverb states, "If a thing is worth doing, it's worth doing well" (though as you can see by the quote at the top of this chapter, G. K. Chesterton thought otherwise). The version of that wisdom that resonates most usefully for me—taking into account the lesson of the clown and my life's experience—goes as follows:

If a thing is worth doing, it's worth doing not so well.

And if a thing is not worth doing, it's not worth doing well.

> *Most things don't have to be perfect. So cut corners if you must, as long as you don't sacrifice the essence or core of the work.*

Chapter 2

An Accident

If, for example, you come at four o'clock in the afternoon,
then at three o'clock I shall begin to be happy.
—ANTOINE DE SAINT-EXUPÉRY, *THE LITTLE PRINCE*

Think where man's glory most begins and ends
And say my glory was I had such friends.
—WILLIAM BUTLER YEATS

When I was very young—certainly less than five—there was a polio epidemic in Johannesburg. It is difficult for people born since the development of the polio vaccine to imagine the overwhelming fear—even panic—that people felt toward this crippling disease. Magazines and papers published scary articles almost daily, often with photographs of children doomed to live in an "iron lung." The frightened mothers of Johannesburg were told by their doctors to keep their children away from other kids while the epidemic raged—unless the children had already been playing together. I had one friend at that time—my cousin Derek—with whom, luckily, I used to have regular playdates. Our mothers determined that he and I would wait out the epidemic together.

Derek had a grand house. A long drive flanked by poplars led up to a large, paved parking area. The house itself had two levels, which was unusual in Johannesburg, where almost all the houses were ranch style. There was a swimming pool too—again not common, far less pools like this one, which had a fountain burbling in the middle. The house even had a terraced garden, the only one of its kind I can remember seeing in all my childhood. When I later learned that the Hanging Gardens of Babylon had been a wonder of the ancient world, it was Derek's garden that came to mind. When I read Hans Christian Andersen's story "The Swineherd," which is set in the palace gardens, I could visualize the swineherd at the bottom of the garden enticing the princess to let him kiss her in exchange for his music box—and I could understand how she might have believed she could get away with it, surrounded and shielded by her handmaidens. She didn't realize that when you are in a terraced garden, whatever you do on a lower terrace can plainly be seen by anyone on an upper terrace.

Derek had a sandbox—much like the one I had—except that his mother had given him baking tins from her kitchen so that he could make sand cakes. He showed me how: You put dark sand at the bottom of the tin and lighter sand at the top. Then, when you turned the tin over, voilà! A ginger cake. I was impressed.

Not all our games were so sedate, however. Derek had older brothers who had gotten hold of some old circular metal casings containing ball bearings. Someone had discovered that if you laid the casings flat on asphalt and swung an ax at them, sparks would whiz in all directions. It was like creating your own sparklers, with the added thrill of swinging the ax, feeling the satisfying thud of metal on metal, and seeing the sparks explode, apparently out of nowhere. So what if some of the sparks hit my naked legs, causing little gouts of blood to trickle toward my ankles! They stung only a little, and it was well worth it. None of us gave any thought to the possibility that the sparks could just as easily fly into our eyes or some other unforgiving part of the body. After all, the sparks seemed to behave themselves. They stayed close to the ground, so why spoil the fun with worry?

In due course, as we might have guessed, some adult took away the ax and sent us to clean up our legs, and someone put Mercurochrome on them to disinfect the tiny wounds. Strangely, I don't remember getting into trouble. I can't imagine why not. It was an innocent time, I guess. Perhaps our activity was viewed as a childish exploration.

Sometimes Derek came over to my house, a small rambler that didn't offer as many opportunities for adventure. But we improvised. For instance, we discovered that by standing on the window ledge of my bedroom and holding on to the burglar bars, we could pee in a big arc all the way into a wide concrete storm gutter that ran along the side of the house. Peeing lacked the unique joys of swinging an ax, but we knew for sure that the grown-ups would disapprove, so it was fun.

Then we had a better idea. Why not ride down the storm gutter on our tricycles? We could start at the top and careen down to the circular concrete wall surrounding the storm drain. What a wild ride it was— very exhilarating! It was only as I approached the wall that I realized I had no way to slow down.

I smacked up against the wall at full speed, and hurtled headfirst into a boulder, on which I cut my lip and hurt my head. Derek summoned my nanny, Lena, and together (I imagine) they got me to my bedroom and onto my bed. Those hours are a blur to me.

Lena tried to reach my mother at the university where she lectured, my father at his law firm, and one or two other emergency contacts, all to no avail. Derek sat on a chair alongside the bed as, throughout the afternoon, I dozed and wakened. Or perhaps I should say, with the advantage of medical training and fifty years of hindsight, that my consciousness waxed and waned, which is a potentially sinister sign after head injuries. The only thing I remember clearly is that each time I awoke, there was Derek sitting nearby—silent, worried, and present.

MANY YEARS LATER I attended a summer conference in Vermont—one of those events where researchers take over a dorm while the college is in recess. To get away from the cloistered environment of the conference, a colleague I will call Joe suggested we take a drive in his Porsche. I jumped at the chance to escape, to see lush foliage and smell the fresh country air. I had not expected, however, that Joe would zoom through the lanes as though on a racetrack, gunning the motor and skidding at the bends. He met my protestations with reassurances, confident but unpersuasive. He had two more Porsches tucked away back in Maryland, he told me, by way of beefing up his credentials. He loved to race them all on the track and had never had an accident.

Then he said something that struck me as quite original.

"When I was young," he said, "I wondered what would be really fun when I grew up. One thing that turned out better than I would have guessed is racing cars."

What was it, I wondered, that had exceeded my childhood expectations? And then it came to me—friendship. I could not have imagined as a child how much joy would come from my friendships, nor how often I would turn to my friends for help or comfort, and how rarely, if ever, they would fail me. I have since learned that just having a friend sitting beside you can be such a comfort that it actually lowers your blood pressure. But I might have predicted that had I just cast my mind back to Derek, sitting quietly by my side as I lay confused and concussed all that long, hot afternoon. I might have predicted what I have often realized since—that a good friend is someone rather special—someone, as Shakespeare said, to "grapple . . . to thy soul with hoops of steel." I learned that lesson for the first time on the day of the accident, and have relearned it many times since.

> *Your friends are your treasures; take care of them. If all you can do for a friend is simply be there, then do so. Just being there is an act of friendship.*

Chapter 3

Crime and Punishment

The human story does not always unfold like a
mathematical calculation on the principle that two and two
make four. Sometimes in life they make five or minus three;
and sometimes the blackboard topples down in the middle
of the sum and leaves the class in disorder and the
pedagogue with a black eye.

—WINSTON CHURCHILL

John Lennon famously sang that life is what happens to you while
you're busy making other plans. In a similar way, for me, learning
has been what happened when I was supposed to be learning something
else.

In third grade, for example, in Mrs. Z's arithmetic class, I was sitting
in the front row. Mrs. Z had written a series of problems on the blackboard
involving addition and subtraction of three-digit numbers. Now
she was explaining at great length precisely how we should tackle the
problem set, which I already understood. My paper and pencil were in

front of me, and the temptation was too great: I polished off the task before she had finished explaining, and offered her my completed worksheet.

Perhaps, child that I was, I expected her to beam in praise. Instead, her face scrunched into a scowl as she bellowed at me, "When did you do this?"

"While you were talking," I said. (The young are so lacking in guile!)

"While I was talking! How dare you!" she yelled, and brought the ruler that she unfortunately happened to have in her hand smartly down upon *my* hand, several times.

THIS EXPERIENCE WAS totally new for me. My parents and previous teachers were all self-confident people, so such a response was unprecedented in my short life. What was I to do?

My brain divided into three entities, each with its own opinion.

One said something like, *This is ridiculous. Aren't we supposed to finish the project, which is exactly what I have done? So what is she mad about?*

The second understood that I had hurt the teacher's feelings. I could sense the pain and fragility beneath the fury.

The third stepped in and took charge: *Shut up,* it said. *Just shut up. Or say you're sorry. The woman's dangerous.*

TODAY, WE UNDERSTAND that different brain regions are specialized to perform different functions, and it's common to view the brain as several separate computers linked in a network. In retrospect, the entity that took charge of my behavior when Mrs. Z whacked me was probably some sort of collaboration between my amygdala (the brain's alarm center) and my prefrontal cortex (the brain's CEO). We know that the amygdala is designed to get you out of harm's way quickly, whereas the prefrontal cortex is slower and more thoughtful—each part working at a speed that suits its function. In this instance, my prefrontal cortex carried the day, which was certainly for the best.

Of course, I had no concept of these matters back then. Both the personal computer and any detailed understanding of the emotional brain were decades away. Even so, I did have a clear sense of different entities within my mind, each giving different input—a committee of brains. This "committee experience" must be quite common. It even shows up in comic books, when the conscience and the baser desires are represented by an angel on one shoulder and a devil on the other, giving contrary advice. However you describe it, what I had stumbled on was an important aspect of wisdom: It helps to allow the different members of our internal committee to voice their opinions—silently—before we choose the right chairperson to speak or act.

SIX YEARS LATER, my emotional brain must have forgotten Mrs. Z and the ruler. By now I was in high school, sitting toward the back of the class and up against the wall. The lowest panes of the tall windows were frosted to prevent students from looking outside instead of attending to the lesson. Our history teacher, Mr. L, was lecturing about something or other, but I found it impossible to pay attention. Instead, I started my Latin homework so that I would have more time to play after school. No one would know, I thought. Since the frosted glass prevented me from seeing out, I figured nobody could see in either. But I had left something out of my calculations. I had not anticipated—though I had heard such stories from older students—that our headmaster would have nothing better to do than to sneak along outside the windows, darting his head up over the frosted panes at random intervals to apprehend such scofflaws as myself.

It would have been a strange, even funny sight to an outside observer to see a middle-aged man creeping stealthily alongside the window ledge. But nobody laughed when he popped up and shouted, "Rosenthal, what have you got there?" I held up Caesar's *Gallic and Punic*

Wars, cringing as though it were a copy of *Playboy*. "Come to my office at once!" he barked, waited for me to exit the classroom, and led the way.

Once in his office, he turned to confront me. He was a stooped man, his face lined and etched by years of anger. "You are going to get cuts," he said, not specifying how many. (The severity of the punishment was measured by the number of "cuts," so named because of the way a cane cuts into flesh.) Caning was worse if you didn't know how many, because you weren't able to count on how soon it would be over. There in the corner was his cane—the sort of long switch you might pluck from a tree while on a hike. It was irregular, like a shepherd's staff, the bark peeled off to make it more supple.

"Bend over the desk and lift up your jacket," he said.

Then, across my rear end, *Whap!* Pause. I had never realized before how thin my trousers were. *Whap!* I had never been caned before. *Whap!*

The cuts were surprisingly sore, but worse than the pain was the humiliation. Although corporal punishment was commonplace in South African schools at the time, a leftover perhaps of British imperial rule, I remembered my parents calling it barbaric. Somehow, that memory comforted me, even though they were nowhere near. I took comfort also in my contempt for the headmaster himself. But he wasn't finished.

"I'm surprised at you!" he said. "*You*, of all people! You ought to be ashamed of yourself." It was apparently not enough to physically assault me. He had to compound it by shaming me as well.

Once again the committee in my mind began its chatter:

Why should you be surprised? What do you know about me? Should I be surprised at you? No, you are well known to be a barbarian.

"Yes, sir," I said.

"You may go now," he said.

I left seething, both at him and myself. What a coward I had been! I should have told him what I thought of him. Sure, that would have gotten me expelled, but so what? Who wanted to be in a school where such brutality was tolerated, sanctioned—even celebrated?

"I'll give you six of the best," he used to say jokingly, referring to the maximum number of cuts permitted, as though talking about some valuable commodity.

YET I LIKED THE SCHOOL, many of the teachers, and my friends.

Everyone was very kind when I returned to class. Nobody laughed. Several said what a jackass the headmaster was, which helped a lot. Even the history teacher seemed genuinely sorry for me, not the least offended that it was his lesson I had been ignoring. Somehow I settled down and got through the day. When I arrived home and examined the damage in the mirror—torn skin, welts, and bruises—I became agitated all over again. But my parents' fury at "that sadistic megalomaniac," my father's threats to call him up and give him "a piece of my mind," and some Nivea cream helped resolve the bruises to both my psyche and my rear end.

As I thought back on the event, I felt bad that I had been caught so blatantly ignoring the history teacher, whom I liked a lot. He had taught us many interesting things, and never talked down to us. Once when he had occasion to mete out punishment to me (I forget why), he ordered me to memorize Shakespeare's Sonnet 18. I had never encountered a sonnet before, but as I started to do my penance, I responded immediately to its magic:

Shall I compare thee to a summer's day?
Thou art more lovely and more temperate

When I reported back to Mr. L the next day to show him that I had done his bidding, he had no interest whatsoever in checking up on me. As far as he was concerned, the matter was over.

It wasn't for me, though. All these years later, I still remember that sonnet, and its words continue to move me and quicken my pulse:

As long as men can breathe, and eyes can see
So long lives this, and this gives life to thee!

Now, that's what I call an intelligent punishment!

> *It is sometimes wise to remain silent, even in the face of injustice.*

Chapter 4

The Persistence and Fragility of Memory

I remember, I remember
The house where I was born,
The little window where the sun
Came peeping in at morn

—THOMAS HOOD

Most of us remember the house of our childhood. Some of us choose to go back and visit the place, if it still exists, perhaps curious to see whether it still looks the way we remember, or for the memories we hope it will evoke. As an adult, I visited the home of my childhood several times, along with my mother.

In the olden days, the house seemed big enough for my parents, two sisters, and myself, as well as a few servants. It now looked rather small, however, and successive owners had made changes—added the inevitable bathroom en suite (at the expense of my old bedroom), installed closets, changed landscaping. But the bones of the house were easy to recognize, and to me, of course, still special. I remembered how as a boy of five, when the real estate agent came to show the house to prospective buyers, I had pushed my bed against the door to sabotage the sale. (My tactic failed.) I must have liked the place a lot.

Most of us have a sense that time passes more and more quickly as we get older. The house of my childhood was the place where for me time passed most slowly; maybe that's why I loved it so. I recall a birthday—perhaps my third—when the party had been set for three o'clock in the afternoon. The morning passed achingly slowly, till finally afternoon arrived.

"What time is it?" I asked my mother.

"Two o'clock," she said.

"And how long is it between two and three?"

"One hour."

"Is that a long or a short time?"

"Not long," she said—but she was wrong. I knelt on the sofa for what seemed like forever, staring out at the empty garden until, on the stroke of three, the gate swung open and children and their mothers poured up the garden path, bearing gifts wrapped in bright paper.

Over the years of visiting my old house, I observed the changes that were typical for Johannesburg as a whole: higher fences; large, angry dogs trained to bark at strangers. The last time I visited, a middle-aged black woman said the madam was out and she couldn't let me see the house. Then she saw my mother coming up behind me and realized, by the "old lady with the gray hair," as she put it, that I was legitimate.

And the most surprising observation? To me, it was a tall bankshire rosebush growing thirty feet or so into the air, and still displaying the fragile yellow blooms I had admired as a child. My mother had planted it half a century earlier, then nursed it carefully. Who could have predicted that the rose would outlive so many friends and relatives, so many political upheavals? I was left with a curious admiration for its tenacity.

So mindful are therapists of the evocative powers of the childhood home that they have developed exercises using imagery that is specifi-cally designed to carry people back to that earlier time and place. Our hope is to reawaken memories that might be useful in therapy. I once employed such an exercise with Jessica, a lawyer in her mid-fifties, whom I had treated for years for depression and issues stemming from childhood. As she used the cues I provided to travel back in time, she found herself in her old living room, playing with her toys. The most telling aspect of the exercise was unexpected—that she could neither see nor hear anyone else in the house. Where was her mother? Or even a babysitter? She couldn't say. As you might imagine, there was much for us to discuss about the neglect Jessica experienced as she was grow-ing up—important feelings that would have been difficult to elicit with-out that guided tour of her childhood home on the magic carpet of memory.

It was in our family's second home that I witnessed the most impres-sive demonstration of the peculiar properties of memory that I have ever seen, an event that consolidated my desire to study the mind. It all began the day my uncle Leonard disappeared. His car was packed and his wife and four children were ready to drive to their farm in the coun-try, but Leonard was nowhere to be found. He had cashed his paycheck that morning and had not been heard from since.

A coordinated search began: Posters with Leonard's picture were sent to police stations all over South Africa, and newspaper advertise-ments offered a reward for anyone who could provide information lead-ing to his recovery. A week later, Leonard presented himself, carrying one of those newspapers, at a police station some thousand miles from Johannesburg. The man in the picture *looked* like him, he said, but he wasn't sure that it *was* him. He gave as his current address the number and street name of the childhood home he had left some thirty years before. This was the only thread of memory he had.

Leonard was retrieved by his wife and younger brother, to whom he introduced himself politely as though they were strangers. They flew him back to Johannesburg, where he was admitted to a psychiatric hospital and found to have no discernible neurological damage—even though he could retrieve no memories. His doctors treated him with high doses of insulin in the belief that putting him into a coma would restore him to his former self. Whether or not it helped, no one can say.

Gradually, over the weeks that followed, his memory returned, starting with his earlier years and progressing in a linear fashion toward the present. At first he believed he was a child, then a teenager, then a young adult. When his children were finally allowed to visit, he could not bear to see them, as they were so much older than he believed them to be. When he saw his sister, my mother, he wept to find her so aged. And so it went, until his memory had all returned and he was discharged.

The diagnosis was "hysterical amnesia": My uncle Leonard had gone into what is known as a fugue state, a condition in which large parts of a person's past slip out of consciousness. Although fugue states are rare today, they were once quite common, especially during wartime. In fact, such a fugue was central to the successful 1941 novel and subsequent movie *Random Harvest*, about a soldier who lost his memory after returning from the war. Yet by the time I did my psychiatric residency in the mid-seventies, fugues were so rare that one of our lecturers predicted that we were unlikely to see a single fugue in our entire career. In my case, he was right—none, that is, except for Uncle Leonard. I have never heard any persuasive reason why fugues, once common, are now so rare.

During wars, fugues were often triggered by the mingled traumas of shelling and bombing, physical and psychological exhaustion, loss of confidence, and war's pervasive chaos and disintegration. Leonard had distinguished himself in World War II, some twenty years before. Then, after the war, he had helped many of his comrades who suffered from shell shock (essentially what would now be called post-traumatic stress disorder) or combat fatigue, including people in fugue states. But he himself returned home apparently unharmed and in good psychological health.

In peacetime, fugues can occur as a response to overwhelming stress, often preceded by some sort of head injury. In Leonard's case, there were certainly conflicts enough in his work and family life to make it plausible that, unconsciously, he had literally wanted to run away and forget his troubles. In addition, he had injured his head and suffered a brief concussion, with memory loss lasting for about a week, exactly one year before the fugue occurred. From this episode he had supposedly made a full recovery.

Whatever the causes, Leonard and other fugue victims show that it is possible to lose large chunks of memory, then remember them again. Where do the memories go? What makes them vanish and then return? Even after more than a century of study, we have no adequate answers.

Animal research shows that fear in response to neutral stimuli (such as a blue light) can be conditioned and deconditioned. For example, rats exposed to a neutral stimulus (blue light) at roughly the same time as a painful one (such as an electric shock) will subsequently respond with fear to the neutral stimulus alone; the process is known as classical conditioning. If the rats are then exposed repeatedly to the blue light only, without the painful shock, the fearful response will vanish—or so it seems. Later, however, if the animals are stressed over a period of time (for example, if their cage is repeatedly rattled), the specific fear responses return. Once again (even without repeating the initial shocks), blue light triggers fear. Clearly, the conditioning has not disappeared. It was merely lying dormant somewhere in the complex meshwork of neural connections that we call the brain. This phenomenon has led neuroscientist Joseph LeDoux to say that "fear is forever." Isn't it fascinating that memories can come and go in animals, depending on circumstances, just as can happen in people? I witnessed that mystery firsthand with my uncle Leonard.

One thing I should say about memories is that they are not static entities like photographs in an album, but dynamic structures that we tinker with as we pass through life. My colleague Daniel Schacter of

Harvard elaborates on errors of memory in his excellent book *The Seven Sins of Memory: How the Mind Forgets and Remembers*. As he puts it: "In essence, all memory is false to some degree. Memory is inherently a reconstructive process, whereby we piece together the past to form a coherent narrative that becomes our autobiography." These words are a humbling reminder as I set out to relate events just as I remember them, aware that my memories are probably not precisely accurate. I take comfort from knowing, however, that the value in what I remember comes more from what the events have given me than from getting every detail exactly right.

For many people nowadays, a greater concern than erroneous memories are those that are lost, often irretrievably. As the world population ages, Alzheimer's disease and other disorders of memory are becoming increasingly prevalent. Indeed, they threaten to overwhelm our health care system.

When I was young, a favorite pastime was blowing soap bubbles in the bathtub—great big bubbles, up to a foot in diameter. In the wall of the bubble I could see reflected in brilliant detail the gleaming tiles, colored towels, faucets, and other shiny fixtures. As the bubbles lingered on my hand, however, the walls became thinner and the images would fade and disappear. I have often thought of those fading reflections as a metaphor for what happens to our memories as we age, how they can fade or disappear as the nerve cells and fibers that support them lose their vigor and integrity. That's one reason I wanted to write this book now, while memories of times past glow so vividly in my mind.

> *Your memories make you who you are; if you lose them, you lose part of yourself. So use and enjoy them, for they are among life's treasures.*

Chapter 5

Know Your Brain

Know thyself.

—ANCIENT GREEK APHORISM

If I wasn't dyslexic, I probably wouldn't have
won the Games.

—BRUCE JENNER

The ancient admonition to "know thyself" has been around for at
least twenty-five hundred years, and it has been attributed to at
least eleven Greek philosophers. Any statement with that much staying
power must surely contain a great deal of wisdom. Of course, it's easier
said than done. Getting to know yourself is a challenge.

First, you keep changing. The self you were in your baby pictures is
very different from all the selves in your later photo albums—the
schoolchild, the student, the young adult, the middle-aged person, the
senior citizen. Second, your capacity to know changes as you develop.
Psychologists who have documented the stages of cognitive development agree that the older you get, the more you are able to know

yourself (unless cognition declines). Also, in a way, the older you get, the more there is to know (because experience keeps changing who you are).

For the sake of simplicity, I have divided the idea of "know thyself" into two chapters: "Know Your Brain" (this chapter) and "Know Your Body" (the next). We all understand, of course, that brain and body interact constantly.

One problem with knowing your brain is that its contents are hidden—until you learn to decode them by the process of thinking. Novelist E. M. Forster wrote, "I don't know what I think until I see what I say." There's a certain truth to that statement. Thinking gets you only so far; after that, you have to see what the brain says or does in order to understand it.

It is also important to recognize the huge variation in the way the brains of different people work. For example, some people have brains that work about equally well in all ways, whereas others have brains that may work rather well in some ways, but quite badly in others. I turned out to have the latter type of brain.

As we saw when it came to cutting out a cardboard clown, my eye-hand coordination left much to be desired, which turned out to be a stable trait. In nursery school, for example, we were asked to fold a piece of paper into a fan. When I showed my effort to the teacher, she took one look and said, "I have seen better fans in my life." As I looked at the other children's fans, I had to agree. Surprisingly, though, instead of feeling offended, I enjoyed her choice of words, which struck me as novel and witty (though to an adult, it might seem like common sarcasm). In high school, my attempt at making a footstool evoked similar scorn from the teacher. So over time I had to face it: I am better with words than at handiwork.

The spatial problem extended to my sense of direction, which remains poor to this day. As a child, I memorized the names of all the streets from my home to my grandmother's place, which everyone thought was very clever. But now I understand I was merely compensating: I learned the street names to make up for my lack of homing-pigeon skills. Another problem with my sense of direction is that even though I "know" it is lacking, I often forget that when I'm out in the field. So I stride off confidently in a certain direction, often with others in tow, only to discover that I have taken us blocks out of the way. Unfortunately, my son, Joshua, inherited this trait from me. I recall one autumn day when we set out for a stroll in Boston. At first, we were lost in conversation, then simply lost. We had no idea where to turn, but we did not despair, as we were used to getting lost. We just kept laughing at our poor sense of direction until we blundered back to our lodgings.

People who have had certain types of strokes can lose a sense of half their body. As a consequence, they may forget to shave one side of the face, or leave one arm out of its jacket sleeve—without knowing that they are walking around with conspicuous omissions. So not only do they not know *what* they don't know, they don't know *that* they don't know—a condition called anosognosia. In a far less obvious way, I have a type of directional anosognosia: Sometimes I don't even know that I might be going in the wrong direction.

Well, too bad—apparently it is hardwired, just the way my brain works. It was a relief to realize that. Now I simply compensate for it—I take a little longer to study the map, and I make a note of landmarks. And as you can imagine, GPS has been a godsend.

A similar realization came when I studied anatomy, where you have to learn not only all the body's different structures but, horror of horrors, their relationships to one another. As I contemplated this problem, the analogy that came to mind was of taking a pot of cooked spaghetti, dumping it out on the table, and having to memorize where each strand fell in relation to all the others. In contrast to myself, a physiotherapy student at our dissection table seemed to know instinctively where all the nerves and muscle fibers went. She probably could have reconstructed the pathways of all the strands of spaghetti in my hypothetical experiment, and I marveled at her powers. To me, she was the Mozart of anatomy, for whom physiotherapy was clearly an ideal career. Comparing our skill levels was as clear an illustration of how differently brains can be wired as I have ever seen. When it came to anatomy, I concluded, she had found her talent; I hoped that once I got past anatomy, I would find mine.

This life lesson, I think, may be helpful to many people. In the course of my work as a psychiatrist, I have seen many children and adults who are deficient in certain aspects of cognition, but outstanding in other ways. Too often, a tremendous amount of work goes into remediating the deficiencies, while not enough attention is placed on developing their areas of strength—or even brilliance. I'm convinced that remediation is not always the best approach. While everyone needs to acquire basic competence in critical areas, nobody can be good at everything—which is worth accepting. Be sure to nurture not only your (or your child's) areas of deficit, but also your areas of strength. For example, if your child loves music and writing, but hates math and computers, he or she should be exposed to all types of musical experiences and be encouraged to write about them. Of course, everyone needs to know how to reconcile a bank balance, but such a child is unlikely to become an accountant or scientist, so don't try to turn him or her into one.

One part of the brain that is certainly worth knowing is your emotional brain. There are many ways to find out what you are feeling. One surprisingly effective way is to ask someone else. Research suggests that other people can often tell what we are feeling better than we can, probably because humans are so good at fooling ourselves. For example, a husband whose wife has just accused him of being angry might turn red in the face and shout at her, "Me, angry! I can't believe you think I'm angry!" Even a passing stranger, unable to hear what the husband was saying, would probably know he was angry, just from his body language.

In recent years, we have become increasingly aware of the importance of "emotional intelligence," a concept that, like pornography, is harder to define than it is to recognize when you see it. In general, emotional intelligence involves not only being aware of what you are feeling but also understanding other people's feelings and empathizing with them. Regulating one's own feelings and expressing them appropriately are also part of emotional intelligence. People with low levels of these skills are bound to encounter social hardships, as others find them strange or disconnected, while those with high levels of emotional intelligence often exceed expectations that were based on their other skills. Group therapy may help both children and adults who lack emotional skills to beef up their abilities in this important area. Such groups may provide a safe forum for giving to, and receiving from, one another useful feedback.

Although knowing one's brain is important for just about anyone, it is especially important for psychiatrists, who are dealing with other people's thoughts and feelings all the time. When I first entered my psychiatric residency at Columbia, I had a supervisor with whom I met each week. When he asked how I was doing in the program, I complained that everybody else seemed so competitive. "I wonder if you have some difficulties with your own competitive feelings," he speculated gently. "What, me? Competitive?" was my first reaction. Well, I soon realized that of course I was competitive. I had been programmed all my life to compete, and for many years it had served me well. On the other hand, my supervisor had hit the nail on the head: Obviously I had some discomfort about those feelings. Over the years since then, I still enjoy competing, but have also seen that life holds riches that have nothing to do with winning. I could not have reached this balance, however, without owning up to my competitiveness and developing a certain comfort with it.

An important part of "knowing thyself" is coming to terms with the darker traits that we all have. One of my teachers at Columbia (I'll call him Ashley), for example, shared an important personal story that has been of great value to me. Ashley told me how as a student and young psychiatrist, he often felt as though others were achieving more than he was. This realization filled him with painful feelings of envy. In order to ward off this pain, Ashley worked day and night, "to fill my plate as full as their plates were so that I didn't have to envy them." But eventually life became so exhausting for him that the status quo was unsustainable. It was just too much.

"So, what did you end up doing?" I asked him, on the edge of my seat with suspense.

The reply was as simple as it was unexpected: "I decided it was easier to envy them." He felt the feeling, named the feeling, accepted the feeling, and voilà! He felt better.

You might be surprised at how often this sequence works. Try it the next time you have a painful feeling.

There are many routes to self-knowledge and acceptance, but the first step is always the same—simply realizing what is there. There is a great value to simply observing experiences, such as your physical feelings, emotions, or thoughts—without judging them. Then you can begin to know your particular brain—how best to use and enhance it; how to celebrate its beauty and brilliance; and how to understand, accept, and work around its deficiencies. I am reminded of the words of an old love song: "Let's take a lifetime to say, 'I knew you well.'" That's how it is with your brain! So get ready for the adventure of learning about your own brain—and the best time to start is now.

> *Your brain is unique. The better you understand its special qualities—both good and not so good—the more rewarding and successful your life will be.*

Chapter 6

Know Your Body

There is more wisdom in your body than in
your deepest philosophy.
—FRIEDRICH NIETZSCHE

As a boy, growing up in South Africa in the fifties, I suffered from a
serious liability: I was bad at any sport that involved handling a
ball. The game of cricket (much like baseball) requires you to hit a ball
with a bat—but I routinely missed.

The problem was compounded by my name—Norman—which had
been given to me in memory of my uncle, who died on the battlefields
of North Africa during World War II. Norman the elder had been that
rarest of rare birds—a Jewish boy who became captain of the high
school rugby team, a position that gave him instant hero status in the
eyes of the family and beyond. Perhaps, in giving me my uncle's name,
my father hoped that I would somehow magically acquire the elder
Norman's athletic gifts. In this regard he was to be sorely disappointed—
but not for lack of trying.

In one attempt to enhance my cricket skills, for example, my father established a Sunday-morning cricket club in our backyard and invited kids from far and wide to participate. Some have since told me that these Sunday-morning games were a highlight of their childhood. Here is a description by Rod Freedman, a childhood friend with whom I reconnected decades later via Facebook.

> I recall Sunday mornings playing cricket at your place with your very energetic father organizing proceedings in your big back-yard, with your mother putting on spreads for morning tea. Your dad gave me a shilling once for making a spectacular catch—probably the highlight of my cricket career!

For me, though, these mornings were a weekly reminder of my shortcomings in an area that clearly meant so much to my father.

Later, I had just as much trouble with golf, even after my father gave up teaching me himself and hired a pro. Unfortunately, the pro was no more successful. "Feel the head, feel the head!" he cried out in desperation, as yet another divot went flying through the air, while the ball sat securely on the tee. It was a strange expression, "Feel the head," and I had an urge to turn the club around and run my hand over its head, but I knew what the poor fellow meant. He himself clearly had an ability to feel where the head of the club was in space as it curved through its proper arc to hit the ball. Any such "feeling" was alien to me.

This inability to "feel" spatial relationships is no doubt related to my poor sense of direction.

The story has a happy ending, however. As I was being shuffled from position to position on the team, something wonderful happened: I turned out to be quite a handy wicketkeeper (much like the catcher in baseball). For some mysterious reason, as I watched the bowler, I seemed to know where the ball would end up so that I could be in place to catch it. Also, it emerged that when the ball was close to my body, I could catch it quite well—well enough, at least, not to embarrass myself or my poor father. The same skill emerged when I played Ping-Pong; once again, when the ball was closer to my body, I was more able to "feel" it. The lesson here is that if you lack aptitude at one activity, try others till you find something that works for *you*. You may be surprised to find you have hidden talents. In my own case, this lesson has allowed me to enjoy physical activities that don't require hitting a ball with a bat, and luckily there are lots of them.

There were early signs that my son, Josh, had probably inherited some of my physical traits, both good and bad. So I was determined not to pressure him about athletics as my father had pressured me. Nevertheless, when Josh was about eight years old, the whole neighborhood seemed to be enrolling children in the county soccer program. It was billed as a low-pressure way to make friends, learn the game, and have some fun outdoors. So I signed Josh up.

Alas, things did not play out as I had hoped. For game after game, Josh stood on the field, staring into space and rarely approaching the ball. My wife, Leora, and I faithfully turned up for the games, but in retrospect, our presence probably made it all the more embarrassing for him. At the end of the season, even though the team lost most of its games, every child on the team received a trophy—a common charade designed to cushion children from the sting of losing—a quest that seems to me misguided. Everyone *knows* who played well and who did not. Wouldn't it be better to help our children learn to accept reality and deal with it?

That year in our family, however, I think I learned more than Josh did. He hung in through the season, but after it was over, he said to me, "I'm not playing soccer next year—no way! And before you sign me up for anything again," he added firmly, "please consult me first." I was justly rebuked.

My poor eye-hand coordination has often helped me as a psychiatrist, because most of my patients (and most people, for that matter) lack one skill or another in a way that puts them at a disadvantage. Some are disorganized. Others seem to have no internal clock, so they are always losing track of time. Yet others have problems keeping tabs on their money, so they are forever bouncing checks.

The key is to analyze the situation, whatever it is, and find a way to work through it or around it. I try to help my patients understand that we all have strengths and weaknesses; that we need to build on our strengths, while also locating and using whatever help we need to deal with our weaknesses. That might mean finding a coach or, in many instances, simply finding someone else to do the things that you do badly. For example, you can hire a bookkeeper to come once a month and deal with your bills. "It's a lot cheaper than all those surcharges for late payments," declared one of my patients. She has never looked back since getting help with her bills.

Sometimes the coach is already there, as with one couple I treat, who were chronically late because the man had no sense of time. By contrast, his wife was very capable in that respect, but he wouldn't listen to her. By helping him understand and accept that keeping track of time was just one of those things he didn't do well—though he was skillful in other ways—I helped him cede control of their timekeeping to his wife. Now they get places on time, which is much more fun than starting a meeting with excuses.

I have shared stories about my poor eye-hand coordination with some of my patients over the years to help them feel less bad about whatever it is they don't do well. We have laughed together at my klutziness and at the pro who urged me to "feel the head." Little could he know what a gift he gave me in that slogan, or how it would come in handy for so many people.

At this stage of my life, with nothing to prove physically (except to myself) and nobody applying any pressure on me, I enjoy exercising more than ever. Like Frank Sinatra, I do it my way: I go for brisk walks, do yoga, and work out with weights. Nobody cares how well I do. What a relief! The experience has led me to encourage patients to enjoy the use of their bodies at whatever level they can.

As to the message Josh gave me, I heard him loud and clear. Never again did I sign him up for an activity without consulting him first—which has worked out well.

> *Whether you are a champion athlete or a weekend warrior, listen to the wisdom of your body and let it educate you about the nature of strengths and weaknesses, both in yourself and in others. Let your body's wisdom guide you as to what activities you are most likely to enjoy and benefit from.*

Chapter 7

Be Yourself

The Importance of Authenticity

This above all: to thine own self be true.

—SHAKESPEARE, *HAMLET*

Be yourself; everyone else is already taken.

—OSCAR WILDE

In the large courtyard of an art gallery in Naples is a sculpture that looks, at first glance, like a gigantic human skeleton, its white plastic bones gleaming in the sun. But apart from its size, something is off about this skeleton. What can it be? you wonder, as your eyes scan along until you see, reaching far into the clear blue Neapolitan sky, a huge spike rising from the center of the face. The nasal cartilage looks extended—grotesquely so, you think—until you realize to whom this skeleton belongs: It's Pinocchio, the friend of your childhood.

Pinocchio is one of the few stories I remember my father reading to me; he is also the storybook character with whom I most closely identified. He was full of high spirits and courage and landed up in outrageous predicaments. Along the way, he encountered crooks—the Fox and the Cat, who misled and cheated him. My father wore a knowing smile as he read about the Fox and the Cat; as a lawyer, he had seen more than his fair share of crooks, and was wise to their ways.

Not so Pinocchio (or me). Pinocchio always wanted to think the best of people, and he paid dearly for his folly. And then, of course, he was a puppet, manipulated by others. No wonder he lied, I thought. His words were about the only things in his life he could control. Beneath all of Pinocchio's wild adventures and mishaps lay one core desire—to be a flesh-and-blood person, not a puppet but a real live boy.

After my father had finally grasped that I could not be shaped into a reincarnation of his football-hero brother, he found a more promising avenue for his vicarious ambition—my academic achievements. He followed my report card as closely as if it were his own, savoring each A and quizzing me about the B's (How did I let *that* happen?). Then he zeroed in on class ranking. What? I had let *that* girl beat me, *again*? And so on. There was no point in trying to explain away a subpar grade; he tolerated no excuses. "Results tell!" he would declare, putting an end to the discussion.

Over time, though, I realized I did not have to tell him when I had a test. He would get the big picture in time. Nor did I need him fiddling with the day-to-day details. Bit by bit, I learned how to do what I liked and avoid what I didn't. I spent afternoons playing in the yard or hanging out with friends. I read books of my own choosing. In my senior year of high school, I avoided the obligatory morning prayers by somehow managing to get appointed as a monitor, along with a friend of mine. Every morning we'd spend a pleasant half hour patrolling the grounds for kids who were playing hooky (though we never found any).

Our Latin teacher, Dr. T, an Italian woman whom I loved, appointed me to manage the C chess team—the worst in the school—a motley crew with dubious interest in the game. It was a task for which I had no appetite, and I managed to let the team disintegrate. At the end of the year, Dr. T remarked to the class: "That Rosenthal is a genius: When the year began, we had a C chess team. Then we appointed him manager, and now there is no C chess team." I was impressed by her shrewdness in discerning that the sorry fate of the team had been strategic on my part, not simply accidental.

Although I successfully evaded my father's scrutiny of my day-to-day academic pursuits, I did integrate aspects of his value system that turned out to be useful. Even though I already knew that A's are better than B's, his interrogations added a visceral twist to my desire for excellence. I stopped making excuses, even to myself, when I fell short of my goals. Although I would never have admitted it to my father, I inwardly acknowledged that results did matter to me, and that I did indeed want to do as well as I could.

For some reason, in my last years at the school, the headmaster decided to take a personal interest in my education—for example, when he heard that I had decided to switch from taking history, which involved digesting several large tomes, to applied mathematics, which looked a lot easier. I was beginning to appreciate my difficulty in sitting for long stretches with long texts; solving problems in math and science seemed better suited to my abilities. I actually enjoyed solving puzzles. This decision did not sit well with the headmaster, however, who called me into his office.

It was difficult for me to step into that room without remembering being bent over the desk, beaten and humiliated, and that memory did little to make me receptive to his mentoring, which I'm sure he regarded as well-intentioned. He made his pitch for my studying history. "We are producing a generation of technical savages," he declared, "people who are very skillful at making things work but have little knowledge of culture. C. P. Snow said it all in his *Two Cultures.*"

I gave some weak response, like, "I am very interested in culture. I read a lot," which he took as a challenge. "Oh, yes," he said. "Then what is balkanization?"

I took a guess and got it wrong.

"Balkanization is the process of dividing countries up into smaller, mutually aggressive territories. That's what you'd learn if you took history."

He seemed to think he had made his case. I didn't, but I thanked him and left.

Then I signed up for applied mathematics and for the next two years enjoyed learning about the swoops and trajectories of Newtonian physics.

In South Africa we followed the British system of medical training, going straight from high school to medical school. Even though the question of specialization was years away, I'd had a strong inclination to become a psychiatrist since witnessing Uncle Leonard's fugue, and I was outspoken about my interest. That idea appalled my father. "I once met a psychiatrist in Howick," he said (referring to a small South African town that almost nobody has ever heard of), "and he was certifiably crazy. Crazy people become psychiatrists, or psychiatry drives them crazy. Either way, it's not for you. It's the rear end of medicine." It was hardly worth commenting on the anatomical incorrectness of his statement, though he repeated it several times to make sure he'd been heard. Even my mother, who normally let me run my own life, weighed in on this one. "Why not go for some other specialty?" she asked. "Like what?" I said. "How about pathology?" she suggested, picking a specialty that had never once crossed my mind as being of interest to me.

Since both my parents had visions as to what I should *not* become, it was particularly important for me have a vision of my own. Luckily, I had no doubt that I wanted to become a psychiatrist, and it is one decision I have never regretted. As Confucius said, "Choose a job you love, and you will never have to work a day in your life." That's pretty much how I feel about my own work, at least most days, and for that I am very grateful. I am also grateful that once my parents saw that my mind was made up, they supported me in pursuing my goal. Not all families do, and I have seen how destructive that can be.

Two asides: If you are a young person at odds with your family in this way, it may be helpful to find other adults (such as teachers, members of your extended family, and parents of friends) who will support you in your goals. And if you are a parent in this scenario, it's worth considering that people seldom succeed at things they are forced to do. Extreme examples of this include a few people I know who went all the way through medical school, only to decide they didn't want to be doctors. One of these young people handed his parents his diploma on graduation day and said, "Here. I've done what you wanted me to do. Now I'm going to do what I want to do." And he walked away. Bottom line: In most cases it makes sense to let your children choose their own careers.

One small caveat about "being yourself": I have come across several people who take this philosophy to a maladaptive extreme. For example, one young employee in my organization said she "wasn't comfortable" being told not to leave the front desk unattended, even though that was part of her job description. Many of us dislike doing things that we have to do in order to accomplish our goals, but we grit our teeth and do them nonetheless. Several subjects in my medical school curriculum, like ear-nose-and-throat surgery, fell into that category for me, but they were requirements for graduation. In today's tough job market, many people have to work extra hours, and telling your boss you don't want to do a part of your job or that you need more "me time" is unlikely to be well received. In fact, even in the best of times and the most congenial of jobs, there will always be some dull, tough, or unpleasant patches. So part of being yourself involves enduring discomfort or delaying pleasure so as to accomplish your larger goals.

MORE THAN HALF A CENTURY has passed since my father read Pinocchio to me at bedtime, and like Pinocchio, I have crossed the sea. I have tangled with the equivalent of the Fox and the Cat (see chapter 32). I have had my full share of adventures. But it has been a long time since I felt like a puppet on a string, forced to live my life so as to fulfill another person's dream. Sometimes I still think of Pinocchio, waking up in his bed and discovering he is a real live boy at last.

I know how good that feels.

> *It's a great comfort to be yourself, and a goal worth striving for, even though it may temporarily make life more difficult.*

Chapter 8

The Weight of History

To be ignorant of what occurred before you were
born is to remain always a child.
—MARCUS TULLIUS CICERO

Although I opposed our headmaster at the time, in some ways I have to admit he had a point. There is no escaping history. It shapes our lives. Here is how it shaped mine.

I grew up in a Jewish community in suburban Johannesburg under the influence of two huge historical forces: the Holocaust and apartheid. Like the force of gravity, their influence was powerful and ubiquitous, even when it was not directly visible.

The term "Holocaust," is derived from the Greek words "whole" and "burnt," and means "everything burnt"—a fair description. The word was not in wide usage when I was growing up; I first heard it when I was in my early teens. Until then, my parents referred only to "the killing of six million Jews."

To me as a child, the Holocaust seemed far away and long ago—though, in fact, it had ended only five years before I was born. In part, that remoteness may have come about because both my parents were born in South Africa, and my grandparents had come to the country when they were very young. So no one in the immediate family had experienced the horrors of Nazi Germany directly. Yet the impact on them must have been enormous, and I did hear the stories. My mother's father, for example, had lost most of his eleven siblings in the killing fields of Lithuania.

We were told that one of these siblings, his brother Tzadik, had died a hero's death: He had killed a Lithuanian guard and a Polish commander with his bare hands, saying, "If I'm going to die, so are you." Yet if I thought about the Holocaust at all, my mental picture was static and remote, like a scene in a snow globe.

Years later, however, Leora and I were visiting London, and my cousin John showed us an eyewitness report of Tzadik's courage. It was a beautiful day, of a kind that is unusual in England and therefore appreciated all the more; we were sitting outside a pub, enjoying the sunlight. But as I read the story of Tzadik's brave death, tears began to roll down my cheeks. Only then did I appreciate how the traumas of a person's family history are implanted in the heart, exerting their silent influence, and waiting to pour out when the right switch is thrown.

At school, the father of one of my friends, an official on the board of education, used to come and address the students periodically about the Holocaust. "From the camps, people would send their friends postcards with roses on them, saying, 'Come; it's good here.' It was all a ruse to get more Jews to the camps without making a fuss," he said, breaking down in tears. Whatever the text of his speech was, he always seemed to wind up weeping. Our reaction? We were embarrassed, especially my friend.

With the benefit of age and experience, of course, I understand that there was much to cry about, and also that my bland reaction to the stories was technically "dissociation," a kind of numbing that people often experience in the wake of trauma. It's one way the mind and body cope: When we are injured beyond endurance (or experience such injury in those close to us) either physically or psychologically, internal opiates kick in to relieve the pain. I have seen such responses many times in my practice, and literature is replete with examples of dissociation, like this passage from Charles Dickens's *Hard Times*:

> "Are you in pain, dear mother?"
>
> "I think there's a pain somewhere in the room," said Mrs. Gradgrind, "but I couldn't positively say that I have got it."

FOR AN EXAMPLE of psychological dissociation in literature, you can do no better than Lady Macbeth. Having urged her husband to kill the king, then helped him to do so, she muses sometime later, "Yet, who would have thought the old man to have had so much blood in him." She distances herself from the horror of what she has done by focusing on an incidental detail—the amount of blood spilled.

So it was with me and the Holocaust. In a sense, I was a Holocaust denier. I knew it had happened, but I denied its significance to millions of people, myself included, and I'm sure there were many others like me. I think my family and others just wanted to put the horrors behind us and get on with our lives. To do so we minimized the impact of this massively important event. My family boycotted German goods, as did many other Jews, and did not want to hear a good word about anything German. Aside from that, though, our focus was on the present and future.

In the Jewish school I attended, everyone in class must have had some stories to tell about how their own family had fared in the Holocaust. Yet nobody asked and nobody told. I feel sad when I think of the lost opportunities. We could have learned so much from one another, including how to offer empathy and support.

The magnitude of this loss came home to me as members of our class became reacquainted via Facebook almost fifty years after graduating high school. One of my former classmates, Lucille Berro, shared with me the history of her family—an extreme example of the type of story many of us must have carried, but seldom if ever mentioned. Lucille, a rehabilitation therapist now living in Australia, is a Sephardic Jew (meaning that her family had lived in areas that fell under Spanish rule and spoke Ladino, as opposed to the Ashkenazi Jews, from Eastern Europe, who spoke Yiddish). Her parents grew up on the Mediterranean island of Rhodes, to which their forebears had fled in 1522 to escape the Spanish Inquisition. The Jews of Rhodes were among the last to be rounded up by the Nazis in the final years of World War II. Lucille's mother, Sylvia, along with her aunts and uncle, were among the last prisoners to enter the death camps. (Lucille's father had escaped from Rhodes earlier.)

What became of Sylvia and her family is an all-too-familiar story: starvation, freezing, filth, lice, harsh working conditions, and ultimately, for most inmates, death. Sylvia herself escaped the gas chamber on three separate occasions, each time by sheer luck. The first time, she was in the sick bay with measles. The sick bay had been cleared out just two days before, its inmates carted off to the gas chamber, so it was not due to be emptied again just yet. In the meanwhile, as Sylvia languished safely in the sick bay, the inmates of her former barracks were sent to be gassed, including a sister whom she never saw again.

I have encountered many such stories of narrow escapes in tales from the Holocaust, including that of Viktor Frankl, whom I discuss in chapter 46. But even apart from the death camps, there's often a roll-of-the-dice quality about who lives and who dies. A friend of mine who interviewed survivors of 9/11 met a man who would have died that day, except that he'd had to take his dog to the vet. It was, my friend observed, ironic that whether a person lives or dies could hinge on the health of a dog.

On the occasion of her second escape, Sylvia had actually been taken to the gas chamber. If business had proceeded as usual, she would have died a horrible, suffocating death. For you to understand what *actually* happened, however, I need to explain that the gas chambers at Auschwitz were partly manned by Jewish inmates called *sonder-kommandos*, who would (after some time) themselves be executed. There was a significant resistance movement among the sonderkommandos, who had managed to smuggle explosives into the camp. At the moment Sylvia was waiting in the gas chamber, these sonderkommandos rebelled, attacking the SS guards and blowing up a crematorium. Sylvia had escaped death by gas for a second time.

Sylvia's final last-minute reprieve occurred on May 8, 1945, in her last concentration camp—Theresienstadt. She had been due to be gassed that very week, but Russian soldiers liberated the camp in time. Instead of death, Sylvia received black bread and thick soup—the first thing that resembled a proper meal in more than nine months.

This woman and her family, which included my classmate Lucille, were the only Sephardic Jews in Johannesburg, where the Jewish community consisted mostly of Ashkenazi Jews from Lithuania. As such, she and her family felt very much alone. When we connected on Facebook, Lucille wrote to me, "We used to chat to each other quite a bit in class. I remember one day you said that I looked like the Mona Lisa. Do you remember that at all? I didn't really know what you meant by it, but I took it as a compliment anyway." I don't recall the exchange, but I do remember her lovely half smile—kind and enigmatic at the same time—so it sounds like something I would have said. Her comments made me wish I had reached out more to her and others. Lucille and I spoke via Skype not long ago. We had not seen each other in forty-five years, but I would have recognized her anywhere. The conversation was full of warmth and, despite our not knowing each other well, of love born from our shared past. At last, with distance and time, the dissociation of my youth has slipped away, and I am able to feel more intensely, both the horror of the past and the joy of the present.

OF THE TWO HISTORICAL FORCES that most directly shaped my growing-up years, the first (the Holocaust) had direct bearing on the second (apartheid or, more generally speaking, the South African political situation). Although I hesitate to delve into (and try to simplify) the complex and murky realm of South African history in general and South African Jewish history in particular, I need to fill you in on some basic facts, in order to give you a context for some of the stories that follow.

Many early South African Jewish immigrants had fled the discrimination and pogroms of Eastern Europe years before the rise of Hitler. South Africa had given them safe harbor and more: They were allowed to practice their religion freely, to own land, and to follow occupations of their own choosing. They felt lucky to be there, so it's no wonder that the majority were inclined to mind their own business and not make trouble—an attitude reinforced by events in Europe during World War II. Jews felt a pervasive fear of anti-Semitism, which history had shown could surface anywhere, as it had even in über-civilized Vienna, where Jews had felt fully integrated, safe, and at home. And indeed, anti-Semitism lurked just below the surface among many non-Jewish white South Africans. It was kept in check largely by the far greater division between whites and blacks, and by the government's desire not to further subdivide the whites, who were already in the minority.

As for South African Jews, they found themselves in a novel and morally awkward position. Having been persecuted for centuries in Europe, then having seen their kin slaughtered in unprecedented numbers, they were now well-off. They had the freedom to conduct their own affairs and (for the most part) the means to do so. But this well-being came at the expense of the black majority. It was black South Africans who did most of the dangerous, arduous work that built the country's infrastructure, who mined its diamonds and gold and provided domestic help—all at bargain rates, while being forced to live apart and in squalor. And Jews, having been persecuted, understood their suffering very well. If we were honest with ourselves, we knew we were part of the system. Moreover, the situation was unmistakably getting worse.

My father, a lawyer at the Johannesburg bar, used to boast about South Africa's independent judiciary. Even if that were true, however, a judicial system is only as good as the laws it upholds, and the laws had discriminated against blacks throughout the first part of the twentieth century. Then, in 1948, two years before my birth, the screw tightened: the Afrikaner-dominated Nationalist government was elected into power, along with its philosophy of apartheid. After this turning point, South African laws became increasingly discriminatory, and the rights of all citizens, especially the black ones, were increasingly corroded. The title of Alan Paton's famous novel *Cry, the Beloved Country* encapsulates the feelings that many shared.

When I was growing up, blacks were not allowed to live in cities or in white areas. In order to hold jobs there—as many needed to do— they had to dwell far away from their families, in servants' quarters or primitive hostels, and they needed a document called a "pass." Even with a pass, though, in some areas they were not allowed to venture out after dark without an additional document called a "special." I will not attempt to detail the inequities and indignities that multiplied with every passing year. Suffice it to say that over time, almost every human right was legislated away. Minor infractions could be brutally punished and often were. The country became increasingly a one-party police state that maintained strict control of its citizens by means of fear.

The South African Jewish Museum is an elegant building nestled in the foothills of Table Mountain in the center of Cape Town. Its windows afford the visitor a view of the mountain and the beautiful city. Inside there is a display of a shtetl (little town), typical of the villages from which the Jews of Eastern Europe had come. What struck me most was the re-creation of a typical shtetl home. How tiny it was!—in dramatic contrast to the large homes occupied by most South African Jews.

Another display, which struck me powerfully, featured the voice of Nelson Mandela talking about South African Jews. Mandela acknowledged that Jews had helped blacks in many ways. It was, for example, a Jewish firm that took in the young Mandela for his law articles, a necessary step in becoming a lawyer. Jews had been among the leaders of the African National Congress, the chief resistance movement against the apartheid government. But at the same time, Mandela said, many Jews simply stood by, without opposing apartheid in any significant way.

Certainly most Jews among the people I knew fell into the passive category. The reason was simple: We were all dead scared, and justifiably so. (In chapter 45, you will learn more about my cousin John, who bucked the system to only a minor degree and was tortured for it.) Of course, it was possible to defy the government in very small ways. For a long time the government permitted minor shows of opposition, perhaps because they created an appearance of democracy. But when it came to any speech or act that would seriously threaten the status quo—beware! That was a different story.

When I was ten years old, in 1960, we learned in social studies about the various designs of the huts inhabited by different black tribes—a beehive design for one, a thatched roof for another, and so forth. I didn't find those facts interesting then, and still don't. But something happened that year in our country that was extremely interesting, that you might legitimately have expected to learn in social studies— the Sharpeville massacre. Yet we heard not one word about it at school. The massacre occurred after a band of unarmed blacks protested at a police station in the township of Sharpeville. There is some dispute about how the crowd behaved, but none about how the police behaved: They started shooting. By the time the incident was over, sixty-nine people lay dead and a hundred and eighty were injured, including women and children. Some were shot in the back as they tried to flee.

Years later, my mother described to me how after Sharpeville, she lay awake night after night, afraid for our future. She and my father actually thought of leaving the country, but he was anxious about how he would support the family. Later, in counseling me not to go into law, my father would say, "Law is not a portable profession. It is specific to each country. You need a profession you can practice anywhere." My parents had learned from the Holocaust that you never knew where you were safe. You had to be equipped to leave at short notice. So although they never communicated directly to me their fears about the future, my parents were always clear that someday I would probably have to leave the country.

The same teacher who taught us about the tribal huts also taught us about a day of infamy in Afrikaner history. Back then, it was called Dingaan's Day, named after a despotic Zulu chief. In 1838, a column of six hundred Boers (later known as Afrikaners) fled the hated British and trekked north into Zulu territory. They made a bargain with Dingaan to retrieve some of his cattle in exchange for land. After fulfilling their end of the bargain, the Boers returned to Dingaan's encampment for a celebratory feast. The guests left their weapons outside the encampment as a matter of good form. Soon after the trekkers and the Zulus sat down to celebrate, Dingaan called out to his men, *"Bulala amatagati"*—the Zulu words for "Kill the wizards"—and they promptly slaughtered all the Boers.

It was indeed a day of treachery, justifiably loathed and remembered. But by the time I attended school, numberless reciprocal treacheries had occurred—and those were not taught. The day that had been called Dingaan's Day is still commemorated in South Africa, but it is now called the Day of Reconciliation.

Since my school days, it has occurred to me that the words spoken by Dingaan to his men were the only two words of any tribal language that I ever learned in school: We were not taught the Zulu words for "good morning," "thank you," or "Merry Christmas," only "Kill the wizards—*Bulala amatagati.*" That brings to mind another aspect of fascism: The state controls the message at every level.

It must be much harder for governments to control their message nowadays, since the advent of the Internet and other forms of global communication. But back then, there was no Internet. South Africa didn't even have television until 1971; the minister for posts and telegraphs used to refer to TV as "the devil's box," best suited to disseminating communism and immorality.

So it was that I grew up in South Africa under two dark shadows: the Holocaust and apartheid. I was too scared to oppose the political system in any meaningful way. I grew up with an unspoken conviction that I would someday have to leave my country. I expected a future bloodbath.

In reality, the transition from apartheid to majority rule in South Africa was far less bloody than most people had ever imagined. This outcome was thanks in large measure to Nelson Mandela, a great man, who was regarded as a great terrorist when I was growing up. When Mandela came into power in 1994, he embraced reconciliation rather than revenge, despite his twenty-seven years in prison and the tremendous wrongs done to him and his people.

I recall a cliff side in Johannesburg on which someone once painted in huge white letters: "Free Mandela." Later, someone crossed out "Free" and instead wrote "Hang." This episode is just one small illustration of the divisions that existed in the country. There was in fact a foiled plot to kill Mandela by pretending to spring him from his island prison, then have him shot for "trying to escape." How fortunate for the beloved country that this heroic and bighearted man survived, and that the people embraced him.

> *Understand the powerful forces of history that shape your world. Like a compass to a sailor, such understanding can help you chart your course through life.*

Chapter 9

Mrs. Brown's "Rular"

Imperfections and Limitations in Authority Figures

Have no respect for the authority of others, for there
are always contrary authorities to be found.
—BERTRAND RUSSELL

To punish me for my contempt for authority, fate
made me an authority myself.
—ALBERT EINSTEIN

t was the 1950s—a time of innocence. That was when young people
believed in the authority of adults!—before we were told not to trust
anyone over thirty, before Mrs. Robinson seduced Benjamin, before the
times, they were a-changing. We believed. But then, into this idyllic
picture came Mrs. Brown, a substitute teacher for our third-grade class.
She was pretty, blond (unusual in our all-Jewish school), and pleasant.
She taught us many new things, including how to spell the classic
instrument of linear measurement: She spelled it "rular."

When my parents pointed out the misspelling to me, I could not believe it. Surely not! Surely it was impossible for a *teacher* to misspell a word! Yet she had—a fact I verified the next day when I pointed out her error to her.

My parents were amused by the episode, and when their amusement continued for what seemed like too long, I realized they were laughing not simply at Mrs. Brown for her error, but at me for my naïveté. They thought it was comical that I thought adults were always correct.

This incident had a wonderful effect on me. The comparison that comes to mind is how a physicist might feel if something suddenly fell upward instead of downward. It would throw the whole theory of gravity into question. That's what Mrs. Brown's "rular" did for me. Now that I had proof that an adult could make a mistake—and a teacher, no less—I knew that *any* adult could be wrong about . . . almost anything.

I began to look around for evidence to support this new and enjoyable thought, and indeed, there was no shortage. The Jewish dietary laws were a good example: My mother separated cutlery used for dairy products from cutlery used for meat (sort of). Mistakes abounded and were winked at, though an appearance was maintained that the system was intact. Shellfish and pork are both unkosher—verboten. Yet my parents ate shellfish when dining out. But pork?—never! Under no circumstances!—unless you needed pork products to save your life. My father was heavily critical of any Jew who ate pork, as were many others. But why? When asked why pork was worse than shellfish, one rabbi explained that pigs were unkosher for two reasons (they did not chew the cud *and* did not have cloven feet—both of which are necessary in order for meat to be kosher), whereas shellfish failed the test on only *one* ground—they lacked scales. Such explanations had a hollow ring, as though they had been concocted after the event to explain something illogical.

On reading *Alice in Wonderland* as a child, I was struck by the following excerpt from a mock trial, a brilliant caricature of the type of post hoc reasoning that seemed to abound in the world of grown-ups:

At this moment the King, who had been for some time busily writing in his note-book, called out, "Silence!" and read out from his book, "Rule Forty-two. All persons more than a mile high to leave the court."

Everybody looked at Alice.

"*I'm* not a mile high," said Alice.

"You are," said the King.

"Nearly two miles high," added the Queen.

"Well, I shan't go, at any rate," said Alice; "besides, that's not a regular rule: you invented it just now."

"It's the oldest rule in the book," said the King.

"Then it ought to be Number One," said Alice.

I liked Alice. She was clever and logical, and she stood up to authority—all qualities I admired. In a similar way, my own questioning of authority continued.

The Bible also lent itself to such questioning. I wondered (as many have done) how God could ask Abraham to sacrifice his son, Isaac. I know He gave him a last-minute reprieve (and perhaps had never intended that the sacrifice occur), but even so, wasn't that cruel? How would a father feel, ordered by God to kill his beloved child? Surely that would be a kind of torture! Several other passages from the Bible led to similar questions in my child's mind. Later, when I read the works of Bertrand Russell and others, I realized that many had passed this way before me.

My mother had a simple way of explaining the variations and contradictions in religious practice and sacred writings. "Everybody picks and chooses from their religion," she said. "They do whatever they want." That corresponds to my own observations, at least for most people.

As for dealing with earthly authorities, we are also in a predicament. On the one hand, we depend on elected officials and other authorities for all sorts of decisions and services, yet every day we read in the newspaper about this or that official who has fallen from grace or failed to deliver on a promise. Also, I suspect that for every miscreant authority who gets caught, many others escape.

Since third grade, however, I have been forewarned to distrust authority figures, and I have Mrs. Brown to thank for that. She might have been the first authority figure in my life to fall short, but she was by no means the last.

> *Be wary of authority figures. They are human, fallible, and powerful—a potentially dangerous combination.*

Chapter 10

All the Lonely People

A Teacher Gives Me a Lesson in Loneliness

The most terrible poverty is loneliness, and the
feeling of being unloved.

—MOTHER TERESA

M s. L, our fourth-grade teacher, was an unusual person. Before en-
tering her class, I had been told by the principal of the junior
school that she was a bit of a drill sergeant, which indeed she was. She
had a ramrod-straight bearing, a wrinkled face, and a basso voice.
"Wipe that grin off your dial!" she would boom from across the classroom, "or I'll make you smile on the other side of your face!" The image
was strange—smiling on the other side of your face—but one you did
not want to explore. It was a sight to see Ms. L striding briskly to class,
her head covered by a helmet of gray curls, diligently puffing away at a
cigarette as though it were one of her official duties.

It soon became clear to me, however, that Ms. L was more than a
military parody. On one occasion, when my parents were required to

sign off on test scores, my father decided to lay it on thick. Paraphrasing Churchill, he wrote on my notebook, "On a cold winter's night, this result warms the cockles of an aged parent's heart." Ms. L liked that. "Tell him," she said, not to be outdone in the arena of melodrama, "that I hope that on a hot summer's day, your work will cool his fevered brow." Clearly I was just a go-between in this romance of letters.

Ms. L loved poetry and would recite a poem in Afrikaans in which one of a pair of identical twins describes the relationship between himself and his twin. The two were so close, and their identities so intertwined that when one twin died, the other (the narrator) did not know whether it was he or his brother who remained alive. As the poem ended, Ms. L would tear up, and her voice would become so wistful that I was sure she was recalling something from her past.

But Ms. L's favorite poem was "Meg Merrilies" by John Keats, about an old Gypsy woman who lived alone upon the moors. She had us memorize and recite this poem, and scolded us for not putting enough emotion into our rendition. We students soon learned that there was no limit to how much we could safely ham it up. No amount of fervent vocalization, facial grimacing, or melodramatic gesture was absurd enough to make Ms. L realize that her chain was being jerked. One girl grinned widely as she chanted, "Her wine was dew of the wild white rose," while twirling her arms like windmills. Ms. L beamed on proudly. When Ms. L herself reached the last lines of the poem, she would choke up, her voice full of grief, as though she were talking about a dear departed friend.

> God rest her aged bones somewhere—
> She died full long agone!

It was clear to me—as it may have been to others—that Ms. L identified deeply with the old Gypsy: another proud woman, lonely but strong and self-sufficient. Like the twins in Ms L's other poem, however, one was dead, the other left behind.

The years passed. I graduated from high school, then medical school, and became an intern at the Johannesburg General Hospital. One night, Ms. L was admitted to our ward with a chest infection, a complication of her chronic obstructive pulmonary disease. Her years of smoking had finally caught up with her.

She was very happy to see me, and especially to have me as her doctor. "Your father must be so proud of you," she said. She reminisced with me about my old class. "Remember Elan Green," she said. "He was so pretty—too pretty to be a boy, really."

Ms. L's illness persisted for days. No visitors came. The medical team, diligent under any circumstances, worked extra hard with her because they knew she had been my teacher. We gave her antibiotics, steam inhalations, and oxygen. The physiotherapist turned her on her side and clapped her chest wall to help her cough up infected sputum. I would stop by and chat whenever I passed her bed. Sadly, our efforts were all to no avail. She succumbed to the infection.

FOR ME, THE LIFE OF MS. L was an early lesson in loneliness. We humans—like all primates—do best in families and groups. So even though Ms. L. soldiered on and had much to be proud of—I was just one of hundreds or thousands of children whom she had educated— hers was a sad lot, bravely borne.

The title of this chapter comes, of course, from the Beatles' haunting song "Eleanor Rigby." How curious it is that at the meteoric height of their popularity, this legendary group could sing about "all the lonely people."

Recently, I was reading an interview with another pop icon, Lady Gaga, who has chosen bullying as a special cause. What can an individual do to counter bullying? the interviewer asked. Lady Gaga responded with a simple suggestion: Just reach out to one of the kids who isn't considered the coolest in your class and tell her you really like the T-shirt she is wearing. Her message, which I think is a good one, is to reach out to people who are isolated or lonely—whatever the reason—and help them feel part of the group. Try to be sensitive to those who are outside the mainstream. That is the most important lesson I learned from Ms. L—that, and a love of poetry.

God rest her aged bones somewhere—
She died full long agone!

> *Reach out to those who are lonely, sad, or different, who may be suffering more than you know. As little as a smile or a friendly word can make a difference—and it may make you feel good, too.*

Chapter 11

Lena and Lucas

Old Injuries; Hidden Fears

When I was young, I used to admire clever people.
Now that I am old, I admire kind people.

—ABRAHAM JOSHUA HESCHEL

Lena and Lucas were long-standing family servants. They stoically bore all the burdens and pains of apartheid, some known to me, but many others that I can barely imagine. Even in the context of those burdens, however, they harbored personal and specific pains and fears—just as we all do.

They were as different in temperament as it is possible to be. Lena was a woman of few words, with a surly disposition. Lucas, however, had a face that readily broke into a grin full of mischief, an impression reinforced by a gap where his upper front teeth used to be.

Our house was separated from the servants' quarters by a court-yard, across which washing lines were stretched—a common feature of the houses in suburban Johannesburg. Wet sheets and other laundry hanging from the lines provided yet another buffer between the whites in the main house and the blacks in the servants' quarters.

We children were supposed to stay strictly away from the servants' quarters, which, of course, made them all the more intriguing. From time to time, I would sneak up there (by invitation) and warm myself by the coal fire on which they cooked. I would peek into their small rooms, curious because the beds were set unusually high off the floor—probably to make room for storage, though some said that it offered protection from the Tokoloshe—a powerful small man with fierce teeth who might come for you in the night and bite off your toes if you slept too near the ground. I breathed in the smell of camphor and marveled at an ingenious contraption—a cord strung over a pulley and attached to the light switch—that enabled Lena to turn off her light without getting out of bed.

The windows were small and high—too high to offer a view and too small to admit much light. Like the courtyard, the window height was prescribed by code, written to enhance the separation between blacks and whites. The specific intention behind the small, high windows—though it was rarely discussed—was to prevent anybody from looking in the window and getting lewd ideas.

When our son, Josh, was about three years old, we visited my family in Johannesburg, and he ran across the courtyard as though it were no barrier at all, darting right into the servants' rooms. They were delighted, commenting that he was not like a South African child. He hadn't absorbed the racism that was endemic to daily life there.

MY MOTHER KNEW that Lena ran a *shebeen* (an illegal brewery) out of the backyard. Men mostly, but also women, arrived at all hours and left with paper bags containing, presumably, the local home-brewed beer made from sorghum. For the most part, my mother let the business proceed unchecked. The customers were well behaved, and I cannot recall a single incident in which anyone caused a disturbance.

On one occasion I said something to Lena and must have stumbled over my words, because she flew into a rage such as I had never seen before. Since she was so often silent, I had not realized that she had a stammer, though my mother, a speech therapist, confirmed that to be so. When I stumbled over those words, Lena apparently thought I was mocking her. In her fury, she shouted, "When you have your firstborn, I hope he is unable to speak at all!" Never before had I heard such hateful words from her, nor ever since. I understood at once, however, that she had felt wounded. I apologized and explained that I had no intention of mocking her, and she immediately knew that to be true and rescinded the curse.

Lena suffered many tragedies in her life, including the death of an adult son. She began to consume more and more of her own merchandise and sadly declined into a state of chronic alcoholism.

LUCAS HAD NO INTEREST in alcohol. His specialty was *dagga*, the local word for marijuana, which grew profusely in South Africa. On one occasion, my aunt proudly showed my mother the "delphiniums" growing in her backyard, which turned out instead to be a rich crop of the prized herb.

One day a white policeman came knocking on our door and informed my mother, "Your boy is selling *dagga* out of this house."

"That is impossible," said my mother, with her customary authority.

"No, madam. It is correct. We've had reports that it is coming right out of the kitchen."

They were at that moment standing in the alleged crime scene, where Lucas was staring anxiously at a box on a high shelf. After a while the policeman became suspicious and snapped at Lucas, "What's in that box?"

"Nothing," Lucas said.

"Get it down, boy," said the policeman.

"I'm not your boy," said Lucas. "If you want to get it down, call your own boy to do it."

This kind of truculence from a black servant to a white policeman was almost unheard-of, so much so that it reinforced the policeman's suspicions. He called his own "boy" from the car, who hauled down the box, which turned out to contain nothing other than lightbulbs.

Realizing he'd been played and made a fool of in front of the white lady, the policeman turned to Lucas and said with barely suppressed fury, "I'll be back, and next time, I'll get you!" He left in a huff, his assistant in tow.

Once they had gone, my mother turned to Lucas and said, "Where is it?"

Lucas slid aside a bread tin, which was near where they had all been standing, exposed a hole in the wall, and removed a brown paper bag.

"I don't want to see it again or hear anything further about it," my mother told Lucas sternly, and as far as I know, she never did.

Later I hunted Lucas down and said to him, "Tell me, Lucas, what does *dagga* do for you?"

He gave me his mischievous smile. "It gives you the knowledge of wisdom," he said. By the way the line rolled off his tongue, I could tell it was a familiar sales pitch.

SOME YEARS LATER, my father decided we could afford a swimming pool, and excavation soon began. "What do you need a swimming pool for?" said Lucas. On questioning, it emerged that he could not swim and was scared of the pool. My mother assured him that he would not be asked to clean it, but he remained uneasy.

"You won't need to go anywhere near it," I said, sensing his unhappiness. He shook his head.

As excavations continued, Lucas became more and more withdrawn and preoccupied, and by the time we were ready to fill the pool with water, he had resigned.

When the day came for him to go, we were all sad, as was Lucas himself. He sent a cousin to work for us in his stead, and visited us many times over the years. It turned out that ever since childhood, he had harbored a secret phobia for deep water that no reasoning could shake. He had become convinced that if he stayed on with us, he would die by drowning.

ONE OF MY FAVORITE QUOTES, attributed to both T. H. Thompson and John Watson, is: "Be kinder than necessary, for everyone you meet is fighting some kind of battle." In thinking back on Lena and Lucas, I realize that besides the obvious daily struggle of living in apartheid South Africa, they were fighting their own secret battles of which I was unaware. What I have realized since is that *most* people are engaged in a battle against some sort of adversity. We may never know the nature of the battle, but we don't have to know in order to be tolerant and kind.

> *When a person is rude or unkind to you, consider that he or she may be carrying some hidden burden. What you might interpret as a personal affront may well have nothing to do with you.*

Chapter 12

Lessons from a Fly

Adversity as a Stimulus to Creativity

There is a crack, a crack in everything.
That's how the light gets in.

—LEONARD COHEN

One evening when I was eight or nine years old, I accompanied our neighbor Henry to pick up his children from a party. Although Henry was also a respected lawyer, my father and another of his lawyer friends thought he was a bit straitlaced—stingy, even. As the two lawyers sat in my parents' living room drinking whiskey, the friend remarked on Henry's abstemious ways. "After two whiskeys, he locks the liquor cabinet," said the friend. "I don't like that. I tend to get thirsty." My father nodded in agreement and poured him another drink.

As we sat in the car, waiting, Henry made an observation that, to paraphrase poet-songwriter Leonard Cohen, opened up a crack in my mind, through which the light poured in. It was a moment of revelation.

Henry pointed out a fly in the car that kept banging up against the windshield, time and again, in a futile attempt at escape. "If only he realized the back window was open," said Henry, "he would turn around and fly out the other way."

Henry then went on to compare the fly's predicament to the challenge that pilots had faced in attempting to break the sound barrier. Conventional ways of handling the joystick simply did not work. The man who broke the sound barrier, Henry explained, did so by shifting the joystick in a way contrary to standard practice. That man was Chuck Yeager, who later became one of the earliest astronauts. The problem that pilots had encountered when reaching Mach 1 (the sound barrier) was that the plane would shake violently, as though it were about to explode.

The challenge of breaking the sound barrier was so daunting that another pilot had demanded $150,000 (a huge sum in 1947) to undertake it. Yeager embraced the challenge. Two nights before the planned flight, Yeager broke two ribs in a horseback riding accident. So keen was Yeager not to be dropped from the flight that he sought treatment from the local vet, and told only his wife and a close friend, Jack Ridley, about the accident. It was Ridley who rigged up a makeshift device from a broom handle to enable Yeager to close the hatch of the plane, a normally simple task that his broken ribs prevented him from doing.

The flight went off as scheduled. When Yeager reached Mach 1, the speed of sound and the point at which most pilots instinctively slowed down to avert apparent disaster, Yeager did the opposite: He sped up— and the unexpected happened. As he described it, "I noticed that the faster I got, the smoother the ride." He had broken the sound barrier.

By linking the frustrated banging of the fly against the windshield with the counterintuitive actions that enabled Yeager to break the sound barrier, Henry introduced me for the first time to what has become known as "thinking outside the box." Some think this phrase arose from a widely known puzzle involving a square grid with nine dots arranged in three lines. In case you have never encountered it, I reproduce it for you below. If you don't already know the answer, I suggest you think it over before you read the paragraph on the next page or peek at page 68.

Connect the dots by means of four straight lines without lifting your pen or pencil off the page. The solution is on page 68.

You may find it easier to solve the problem if you copy the 9-dot grid on a sheet of paper.

As you can see, the only way to solve this brain teaser is to extend the lines outside the "box" that your eye creates when you *assume* the solution must occur within the grid—even though nobody told you so.

That's how we often create artificial barriers for ourselves in life. We make certain assumptions about how some problem "must" be solved, and those assumptions can trap us in old ways of thinking. One sad example of this tendency (out of many one could choose) occurs in photo lineups presented to eyewitnesses. At least in the past, police have often asked witnesses whether they recognize one of (let's say) five suspects as the criminal, and witnesses have not routinely been told that *none* of the people in the photos may be a suspect. This creates a bias, made stronger because all Americans, since childhood, have routinely taken multiple-choice tests in which several answers are presented, one of which is correct. Therefore, in the witnesses' minds it may seem natural to construct a mental box around the several photos and assume, based on past experience, that one of the people inside the box must be guilty. So they persuade themselves to pick one. Then, once a wrong suspect is fingered, the police may readily start interpreting that person's actions as suspicious, and an innocent person can easily be convicted.

A more sophisticated term for outside-the-box thinking is a "paradigm shift," a phrase coined by Thomas Kuhn in his famous book *The Structure of Scientific Revolutions*. It turns out that most intellectual revolutions, if not all of them, turn conventional wisdom on its head. A classic example is the Copernican Revolution. Up till the time of Copernicus, it was believed that the sun revolved around the Earth, which seemed obvious. It is, after all, common experience to see the sun "rise" and "set" each day, and this geocentric view of the world is endorsed by no less an authority than the Bible. Yet Copernicus, examining astronomical data, concluded the opposite—and was, of course, correct. That was a huge revolution, but minirevolutions involving small shifts in paradigm occur all the time in science—from which we all benefit.

During my career in psychiatry I have observed several mini–paradigm shifts, and have been fortunate to be a part of one or two

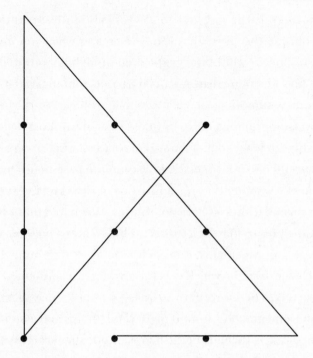

of them. In the last decades of the twentieth century, we saw a major shift in our view of serious psychiatric disorders. We now know that they usually have a biological basis and are not primarily a result of psychological factors, such as, for example, what used to be called a "schizophrenogenic mother." Similarly, in some early work that I did at the New York State Psychiatric Institute, I read through dozens of old charts of bipolar patients, many of whose classic, periodic ups and downs were explained as Freud might have seen them—as psychological defense mechanisms to deal with internal conflict instead of neurobiological fluxes, which is how a modern psychiatrist would typically view them.

Later, after my colleagues and I had begun to study the therapeutic effects of light for seasonal affective disorder (SAD)—another mini–paradigm shift—I discovered a classic case of seasonal affective disorder that had been reported by U.S. Army physician Colonel George Frumkes in 1946. The symptoms were beautifully observed—unmistakable SAD. Frumkes's explanation? The patient's depressions began about the time he learned that masturbation was not a unique sin of his; when there was a decrease in the intense, conscious feeling of guilt. The depression represented a redistribution of the punishment in the psychic economy. . . . There was a megalomanic quality in his identification with the world. . . . He reacted to the onset of cold weather (Mother Earth) as though it were a frustration.

Like the fly bashing its head against the windshield, these psychiatrists did not realize that they needed to fly in another direction. But because they had built their old theories into a large and complicated box, it was difficult for them to think outside of it. No wonder it usually takes years for a new paradigm to dominate a field.

At the time I was planning our very first study of SAD at the National Institute of Mental Health (NIMH), I was still a very junior psychiatrist with an oddball project, few resources, and serious practical problems. For one, the research assistant who had helped me get the study started was a volunteer, who needed a paying job without delay. She couldn't even afford to wait until the experiments were due to begin, so I was desperate. I needed her help, yet I lacked government funds. How could I cover her salary long enough to get us through the winter—the crucial period?

At that time, I happened to be reading one of Freud's famous case studies, "The Wolf Man," about a patient whose real name was Sergei Pankejeff. At one point, Pankejeff ran out of money, but because Freud very much wanted to complete the analysis, he actually lent Pankejeff money to help cover his living expenses. If Freud could lend money to a patient, I reasoned, surely I could pay my research assistant from my own funds—and that is what I did until we could offer her a salary. Considering the importance of the study, it was an excellent investment. But it did require a deliberate shift in thinking.

When my research on SAD was first published, many colleagues thought the concept outlandish, perhaps because it involved thinking differently about people with this new disorder in not one but a few different ways. First, SAD requires thinking of time as cyclical, rather than linear. Previously, a woman with SAD (and her therapist) might explain her winter depressions as caused by reversals of fortune that happened to occur every autumn and winter, followed by strokes of good luck (or the benefits of therapy) in spring and summer—year after year. Second, the idea of SAD involves recognizing that moods can be driven by the revolving seasons, specifically the changing light. Light had to be reconceptualized as more than something that enables crops to grow and people to see, but also as a powerful influence on mood.

It is not only in science but in life itself that we often embrace a paradigm shift—though we don't usually use such a grand term. We may simply say, "I've changed my mind." A man may break off his engagement, for example, because he realizes that his fiancée does not treat him kindly no matter how hard he tries, and it finally dawns on him that he doesn't want to be treated that way for the rest of his life. A woman who has been abused sexually may decide to remain silent no longer and file a complaint. Someone who hates his or her job may decide, "Enough!" and change careers. So it is that by being flexible in our thinking and willing to entertain an opposite set of ideas, we can overcome adversity and improve our chances for success and happiness.

How can we reverse our thinking? First, by understanding that such reversals are not only possible but central to the creative process and even to survival. Second, we may reflect or meditate on a problem until we figure out a new way to see it. Often new insights occur when your state of consciousness shifts—for example, when you dream, relax in a warm bath, or go into a state of transcendence during meditation. Third, we can consult others. And finally, we may derive inspiration from a book—even if that book is a novel, as the following example illustrates.

One of my patients, a brilliant young man, was born with a form of autism spectrum disorder. Navigating his way through the maze of human interactions, which is easy and natural for so many people, was nearly impossible for him. He found a way, however. Growing up, he read and reread Alexandre Dumas's famous novel *The Count of Monte Cristo*. In the novel, the hero, Edmund Dantès, is wrongfully imprisoned in the notorious Château d'If, an island fortress from which escape is almost impossible. Yet escape he does, by exploiting a series of chance events. The first stroke of luck is a crack that appears in the floor of Dantès' prison cell when a fellow prisoner, "the Mad Priest," breaks through in his own escape attempt.

That was the crack that let in the light for my patient. If Dantès could escape from the Château d'If, he reasoned, maybe he too could seize any scrap of good luck and escape from the prison of his mind. Happily, with the support of his family, his own ingenuity, and continued hard work, he has managed to do so and is now working successfully in the world.

I have always found it stimulating to consider alternative ways to view challenges in my life, to find novel routes to attain my goals, to discover the crack in everything that lets in the light. Likewise, in my work with patients, I enjoy helping them look at their life circumstances in different ways, at times exploring opposing options. Together, we think about what has worked for them in the past, and ponder what other approaches might be tried. If we achieve our treatment goals, that's great. If not, I'll say something like, "We haven't figured out the answer yet, but let's keep trying."

Let me end, then, at the beginning—with Henry and the fly in the car. He gave me a great gift that evening: a key insight that would stand me in good stead for the rest of my life. He may not have been generous with whiskey, but he was generous in a way that was far more important to me: He was generous with his ideas.

Try to use difficulties, setbacks, and imperfections as a stimulus to creativity whenever they arise. When you feel trapped, like a fly bumping against glass, look for a novel solution. Fly some other way!

Chapter 13

The Fixer

*My Father's Practical Approach
to Helping People in Trouble*

I try to be the fixer of situations and I gravitate
to people who are institutional misfits.

—STEPHAN JENKINS

I f you were in crisis, my father was a great go-to person. Everybody seemed to know that instinctively, if not by his reputation. If the crisis was embarrassing, you had the comfort of knowing that he would never judge you. His approach was purely pragmatic. His question was always, "How can this best be fixed?" Then he would say or do whatever was needed to make that happen.

Some teachers at our school and their spouses had occasion to call upon my father in this connection. How do I know? He told me, of course—which he certainly should not have done. He regarded it as part of my education, which I suppose it was. To my credit, I respected his confidences.

One female teacher approached my father to say that she and her husband were contemplating divorce. She had met a man with whom the husband suspected she had had an affair. The husband had been a good partner for many years and she did not want to lose him. My father assessed the situation. "*Did* you have an affair?" he asked. She said she had, but it was now over. "You have to deny it," said my father. "Your husband will never accept it and it will mean the end of your marriage."

She took his advice and the couple remained together happily (or as happily as they had ever been) till death did them part.

The husband of a different teacher also approached my father, also with a story of infidelity. As he told me the story, my father, who was an accomplished amateur actor, played the various roles. First, he took the role of the husband—let's call him Louie—walking along the sidewalk, innocently minding his own business. Then my father adopted the seductive look of a woman of the street, beckoning to Louie, who followed like a man in thrall. Next my father became the husband (pimp?) of the woman—delighted to catch poor Louie in a compromising position, whipping out an imaginary camera, snapping several imaginary shots—*pop-pop-pop*. And finally, he portrayed poor Louie again, crestfallen on realizing that he'd been entrapped.

"Have you told Zelda?" my father asked Louie. His terror visible, Louie said he had not. (As Zelda had been my teacher, I could well understand his fear.) "What do these people want from you?" my father asked.

"Money," said Louie. "They say if I give them a hundred rands, they'll go away."

"They won't," my father said. "It will be just the beginning. Tell Zelda everything. Apologize. Tell her you don't know what got into you."

Louie did exactly that, and I'm sure Zelda had plenty to say, but if so, there is no record of it. The bottom line is that she forgave Louie and they also lived happily ever after (or at least as happily as they ever had) till death did them part.

It is tricky to give direct advice even when you're asked for it. Your advice could be wrong, and it is usually best if people can solve their own problems. But my father was a fixer. That's what people came to him for, and in these two instances, it worked out.

WITHOUT NECESSARILY ENDORSING my father's advice, I learned a great deal from these two vignettes:

First, be there for someone in crisis. Don't judge the person at that moment. Judgment is the last thing that a person needs, because shame is very painful. Your acceptance of the person, if not of their actions, will ease that shame. It's like putting balm on a wound. If the action is so reprehensible that you can't deal with it, that's your prerogative. In most instances, however, you may be in a position to help the person and perhaps anyone who was wronged, and to make matters better.

Second, listen well; then customize your advice to suit the situation. While a single transgression—infidelity—was at the root of both dilemmas, the advised actions were quite different. People and circumstances are too complex for any one-size-fits-all approach.

> *Be slow to judge people who are in crisis. If you choose to give advice, be sure to customize it to the people and circumstances.*

Chapter 14

The Long Reach of Sexual Trauma

The past is never dead. It's not even past.

—WILLIAM FAULKNER, *REQUIEM FOR A NUN*

One of the most surprising posts to appear on my Facebook page showed a good-looking young man, seated and posing for a formal photograph. The person who posted the item, a former classmate, identified the man as, let's say J.J., a seventh-grade teacher at our elementary school. Of J.J. my classmate wrote: "He abused little boys for years and the school turned a blind eye to his activities."

The sad thing about this statement is that it is entirely true. It was one of those "secrets" that "everybody" seemed to know and for years nobody did anything to stop. J.J. took eleven- and twelve-year-old boys to movies, his apartment, and on overnight outings to a nearby resort. It was easy to see how people might gravitate to J.J. He was clever, charismatic, sophisticated, and well traveled. He groomed and cultivated his favorites, and those he ignored sometimes felt sad to be left out.

Of the many former students who responded to the post, only one acknowledged that he had been molested by J.J. He reported the event to his parents, and together they took the matter to the principal—who disbelieved the student. The student ended up transferring to another school. The abuser kept his job.

Another former student, whom I'll call Jonathan, described how J.J. used to take groups of boys to a campsite, throw down a ground sheet, and cuddle with his favorites. Even though Jonathan himself was never molested and is a happily married professional, memories of those outings still haunt him all these years later. He points out that J.J. operated with such free rein and impunity that even during class, ostensibly to show an educational movie, he would darken the room and fondle his chosen ones right there in the classroom.

Other children and parents reported these events to teachers and the principal, but were either disbelieved or ignored. It was many years before some rabbi finally got J.J. fired. To my knowledge, this pedophile was never prosecuted.

Responses to these postings flooded in, not only confirming the initial posts, but also voicing—for the first time in a public forum—people's powerful feelings about those events. A few wondered why anyone was bringing this matter up after all this time. It was all so long ago, they thought. Wasn't it time to let it go? As a psychiatrist, however, I have seen how the effects of child abuse can persist for half a century or even a lifetime, and how it is impossible to "just let it go."

Sexual development is so key to the human psyche, and in order for it to develop normally, it is important to be able to trust others—especially those in positions of responsibility—not to interfere with this development. Sexual abuse can derail it, resulting in all sorts of problems—conflicts around sexual adjustment in later life, behavioral problems, and tremendous suffering. The initial poster did well to flag this important unspoken event in the past of so many students who went through our school.

The public policy issue is important as well, but goes beyond the scope of this book. I want to focus here on what my experience has taught me about sexual abuse, especially a few ideas that are not well-known.

Sex Abuse Is as Bad for Boys as for Girls

Back in the fifties and sixties, if anyone thought about the matter at all, there was a widespread sense that if an adult "horsed around" with young boys, it was just one of those things—a sort of rite of passage that one grew out of without any permanent scar. Not so, says psychologist Christine Courtois, author of *Healing the Incest Wound*, who has been treating the victims of child abuse since 1971—and I agree. Courtois finds that abused boys are just as traumatized as girls—though maybe differently. Their passive role in the abusive experience puts them at odds with the socially designated male role of initiating sex, which can create conflict. Abuse of boys by men can create confusion about sexual identity as well, while abuse by a grown woman may be hard for the victim to recognize as abuse. In the eyes of other boys and even the victim, it may seem like he just "got lucky." Over time, however, emotional problems may develop that make it clear that precocious sexual experience is often, in fact, traumatic.

Forget the Word "Willing"

The effects of early abuse of boys is the subject of a 2005 article from the *Journal of Child and Adolescent Psychiatric Nursing* excerpted here:

> While some boys who willingly participate may adjust to sexual abuse, many others face complications, such as reduced quality of life, impaired social relationships, less than optimal daily functioning, and self-destructive behavior.

One criticism that I—and many other clinicians—would level against this otherwise sensible statement concerns the word "willingly." When the person who is the object of abuse is under eighteen, let alone eleven or twelve, the concept of willingness has little meaning, either legally or psychologically. Even between adults, when sex occurs in the context of a major difference in personal power—as can happen in the workplace, the military, and religious and educational institutions—the concept of willingness is highly questionable. If it is hard for adults to say no to sexual approaches from a boss, a commanding officer, the trusted family doctor, or the pastor—as we all know it is—how much harder is such a choice for children?

It Happens with Doctors Too

One of the strangest interludes of my professional career occurred shortly after I started my private practice. In order to get supplementary training in psychotherapy, I sought supervision from a prominent local psychoanalyst, Dr. X. Soon he began to refer to me some of his psychotherapy patients who needed treatment with medications, which was not part of Dr X's skill set. I would call him periodically to discuss the progress of our mutual patients, until one day, out of the blue, he told me never, ever to call him again—and refused to say why. His response to my bewilderment was, "I can't tell you why I can't speak to you for the very reason that I can't speak to you." I was upset, to say the least, as I had looked up to the man. I realized, however, that whatever the issue, it was his problem, not mine.

Sometime later, Joan, a successful professional and one of the women Dr. X had referred, told me that he had made sexual advances toward her in their sessions. Needless to say, such advances would be distressing—not to mention unethical—under any circumstances, but Dr. X's crudeness, coerciveness, and complete disregard for Joan's feelings aggravated the trauma. She was eventually able to break free of the destructive relationship, but declined to take legal action. She believed (justifiably) that any complaint would fail: It would be his word against hers, and she would simply be traumatized all over again.

Years passed and I got a request from the medical board to forward to them records pertaining to Adele, another woman whom Dr. X. had referred to me, who had long since left my care. Shortly after I received the request, Adele herself called me. She hastened to reassure me that the request from the medical board had nothing to do with my treatment of her. Dr. X had sexually abused her, she said, and she was filing a complaint. She told me that Dr. X had become paranoid of me and had accused her of having an affair with me. Finally, it became clear why Dr. X had broken off all dealings with me.

With the permission of both women, I put them in touch with each other so that they could file their complaint jointly and support each other's credibility. In the face of duplicate charges from two credible women, Dr. X immediately, permanently, and irrevocably surrendered his medical license to practice.

The Person Being Abused May Not Know It

One disturbing aspect of sexual abuse (there are many) is the so-called "trauma bond," which may develop during the course of abuse, and which binds the victim emotionally to the abuser. The trauma bond is one answer to the commonly asked question, "Why didn't he or she just put a stop to it or leave?"

One young former prostitute whom I interviewed—I'll call her Annie—told me how she had enjoyed warm and intimate times with her pimp. For example, they would watch their favorite TV shows together, in particular Animal Planet's *Most Outrageous Animals*. She had thought that he cared for her. But later, after some recovery time in a safe house, she was able to get perspective on the true nature of their relationship—one in which exploitation and enslavement masqueraded as affection and intimacy. Later, when she saw *Most Outrageous Animals* on TV, she would have flashbacks and panic attacks and start screaming.

Zeroing in on Trauma Is Not Usually the First Step in Healing

There seems to be a general sense that in order to treat the effects of trauma—such as sexual abuse—you need to rapidly zero in on the traumatic events and root them out. Most experts would disagree, however, emphasizing instead the need for the trauma victim to feel emotionally and physically safe; to stabilize the chaos that usually results from abuse; and to develop an ability to regulate his or her own emotions. This occurs best in the context of a trusting therapeutic relationship. Meditation may also help in this regard. In fact, I met Annie while studying the effects of Transcendental Meditation (TM) on young former prostitutes in Los Angeles, who had been abused multiple times daily while on the streets. TM helped Annie and some of her friends to sleep better and settle down emotionally. Only once that happens can an abused person begin to safely and effectively confront the trauma—and there are several specific techniques that are useful in this regard. A skilled therapist is definitely needed through the whole process.

Silver Linings

So what good, if any, can come from sexual abuse—this particular type of adversity? Psychologist Courtois points out that many survivors of sexual trauma (or any trauma, for that matter) are often more empathic toward other victims, more likely to help them, and generally more spiritually oriented. Like broken bones that knit together to become stronger than they were before, Courtois says, people who have been abused may become stronger "at the broken places." They can become better able to spot potential abusers, set limits with them, and report them. In order to reach this point, however, therapy is usually needed.

One of my patients, Lauren, currently in her late twenties, exemplifies some of these qualities. While attending an exclusive boarding school, Lauren was raped by a staff member. Although she suffered years of emotional aftershocks, with her family's support and psychotherapy, Lauren has succeeded in rebuilding her life. She is happily married with a lovely daughter. She became a child life counselor, working with little children who are so sick that many of them have little prospect of living into adulthood. Tapping into the vulnerability she felt when she was raped, she has been able to reach out to and help some of the most vulnerable members of our society. As part of her volunteer work, Lauren gives talks about her own experience with rape and its aftermath, post-traumatic stress, and her long path to recovery and a happy life.

Many people draw on their own history of suffering, regardless of its specific nature, to help others. For example, one woman I know, who suffered for years from chronic Lyme disease, now spends hours each day on the phone and computer, helping others with the same condition. "I took my illness and turned it into a gift for others," she told me.

It's important to realize, however, that we don't have to experience exactly the same type of suffering as another person to feel empathy and reach out to help. We don't have to catch a finger in a door to understand that it hurts or to empathize with the pain of someone who has done so. Likewise, a personal history of abuse should not be necessary to realize that abuse is a terrible thing.

And if the abuse was not prevented or stopped in a timely way, at least it should be acknowledged. It is just such an acknowledgment that my classmate, who posted the story about J.J. on our Facebook page, sought. And finally, more than half a century later, even though J.J. and all the authorities who turned a blind eye to his activities are long dead, the governing board of the school offered such an apology and undertook to do whatever they can to prevent similar events from ever happening again in their school.

If you or someone you know has been abused, seek out a competent therapist to help heal the wound. Remember also that in the aftermath of abuse, we often see the powerful resilience of the human spirit, as well as our deep-seated drive to convert personal trauma into compassion and kindness, to help others heal.

Chapter 15

Trouble with My Father

Children begin by loving their parents; as they grow older
they judge them; sometimes they forgive them.
—OSCAR WILDE, *THE PICTURE OF DORIAN GRAY*

Not long ago, I attended a conference on the potential benefits of
Transcendental Meditation for veterans with combat-related post-
traumatic stress disorder (PTSD). Several officers in training reported
on their experience with TM and why they had chosen to learn it. One
trainee in particular caught my attention. "I wanted to learn not only
for myself," the man said, "but also for my father, who is suffering from
PTSD."

I could relate. My father also suffered from PTSD (inter alia, as he
would have said—using his legal Latin whenever he got a chance. It
means "amongst other things"). Because of all these other things, it
took me a long time to diagnose his PTSD. In fact, I did so only in retrospect and after his death.

You first encountered my "very energetic" father running around
our backyard, which he had turned into a cricket field, dividing dozens

of aspiring cricketers into teams and offering shillings for spectacular catches. He was given to spells of exuberance, especially as a young adult, which ranged from the hilarious to the ridiculous. He was a gifted storyteller and a flawless mimic. For example, he once managed to wangle free drinks out of an Irish bartender because of his heart-rending tales, told in a heavy Irish brogue, of his sad childhood in Dublin, a city in which he had never set foot. At a Jewish seaside hotel, shortly after the Holocaust, he and a friend reminisced in thick German accents about their days at Heidelberg University (which, of course, neither had ever attended); he regarded it as the ultimate compliment when the people at the neighboring table were overheard telling the waiter to move them as far as possible from "those Germans."

Famous for his wit, my father would often be asked to speak at family gatherings and festive occasions. He also entertained guests invited to dinner. On one such occasion an old family friend brought along Doris, a new lady friend. As was his wont, my father began with jokes that were at first in reasonably good taste but became increasingly off-color as the meal progressed. And my mother, as was her wont, tried to intercede. "No, Charles, not that one," she protested. "Oh, let him, Esta, let him," the lady friend pleaded. "Don't interrupt, Doris," said the family friend. "It's all part of the act."

Dad was not good at answering questions about himself. For example, when I asked about his law practice, he would say he didn't want to bring his work home. I do recall, however, when I was just a boy, one worrisome case of his that went to trial. That evening he came home looking glum and said, "Justice was not well served today." "I'm sorry your client lost," I said, to which he replied, "No, he won."

Charles Dickens would have enjoyed my father for his complexity and eccentricities. My father, in turn, loved Dickens, and identified with the character in *Great Expectations* known as "Aged P" (short for aged parent), an appellation he often appropriated for himself, as in "Give Aged P a hug." Dad was in no way aged at the time, so his choice of this nickname conveyed both the self-dramatization and self-pity to which he was prone. Likewise, he would sometimes say, when he failed to get his own way, "I am treated like a dog in this house. Woof! Woof!"

Dad loved neologisms—newly coined words—and curious phrases that he would pick up here or there, modify, and then assign new meanings. He developed quite a lexicon, and everyone in the family knew it. Indeed, some of these expressions have even carried across the generations. An example: He once saw a B-grade horror movie, *The Naked Jungle*, in which the hero and his mail-order bride are attacked by army ants, called Marabunta, that threaten to devastate the hero's plantation. Everyone in the movie is terrified of "the dreaded Marabunta"— understandably, given their destructive powers. From that time on, my father referred to all types of frightening infections as "the dreaded Marabuntu," altering the strange word so that it sounded more ominous. The phrase stuck, and even today, if Leora, Josh, or I have some type of unpleasant viral infection, we might say that we are suffering from "the dreaded Marabuntu," so keep your distance.

My father was extremely superstitious and adhered to many rituals that most people have never heard of. In fact, existing superstitions were not enough for him. He had to invent some of his own. An example: As he grew older, he developed the belief that even numbers were good and odd numbers bad, and he tried to arrange his world accordingly. When he climbed a staircase, for instance, he always tried to use an even number of paces. If by chance he had used an even number of paces to reach the next-to-last step, he would take the last tread in two little mincing footfalls to ensure that the final number came out even.

In ancient times, there was a widespread belief that when a person sneezed, the devil briefly entered his soul. It is for that reason that even today, when people sneeze, others say, "Bless you," or *"Gesundheit."* An equivalent expression exists in virtually every language. Another superstition requires that the sneezer give his earlobe a tug. I can almost see how, in a person's imagination, pulling the ear might open a trapdoor through which the devil is jettisoned. Well, in my father's case (as you might have guessed), *both* ears had to be pulled, boosting the power of the remedy with the even number. "Pull your ears," he would say, when one of us would sneeze, and he would be quite distressed if we refused. Now, if you were to challenge my father on the reasonableness of these actions (though we rarely did, as there was no point), he would acknowledge that they were superstitions. So he was not delusional, just compulsive.

One positive outcome of Dad's strangeness is that it gave me a life-long appreciation of eccentricity, which has served me well as a psychiatrist. Rather than seeming peculiar, quirky behavior usually interests me, and I wonder how the quirks came about and what benefits, if any, they confer on their owner.

Unfortunately, my father's witty and eccentric qualities were only one aspect of his complicated personality. As he aged, Dad became increasingly irascible and nasty, especially after a few drinks. Although he had a Scotsman's passion for whiskey, he had the liver enzymes and stomach lining of an Ashkenazi Jew. The resulting combination of ill temper and indigestion made him spiteful, and spoiled many an evening meal.

Over time, Dad's predominant affect became anxiety. He worried constantly about money—even though he always had enough. Paradoxically, he was generous to a fault and regarded stinginess as the worst of all human traits. "Be careful of charming people," he advised. "They are bound to be stingy, because charm costs nothing." Though well regarded in his profession, he fretted about his legal standing. Later, diagnosed with diabetes, he worried incessantly about his diet. The trend was downward: Over the years he changed from being good company into someone who was hard to be around.

I had a key insight about Dad on reading Art Spiegelman's brilliant graphic book *Maus II: A Survivor's Tale*. The book is based on the true story of Spiegelman's father, who survived imprisonment in Auschwitz during World War II and later settled in the United States. Using cartoon animals, it depicts the traumas of life and death in Auschwitz, the difficulties adjusting to normal life afterward, and the problems faced by the children of Holocaust survivors. Spiegelman's father reminded me of my father, and the discomfort that Spiegelman experienced mirrored my own discomfort at being around Dad in his later years. Yet Dad had not been in a death camp. So how was I to understand this similarity?

Only then did I set about constructing a coherent narrative of my father's traumatic experiences and their consequences. Why did it take me so long? One reason, I believe, is that severe trauma disorganizes how a person views his own life story. One path to treating trauma is to help a person reconstruct that story coherently. What were the traumas? How did they affect the person? What were the consequences? Sadly, my father never had the opportunity to organize his own life story. Nor was I able to do so in his lifetime. Nevertheless, it seemed worth doing even after his death. I wanted to better understand this complex and mercurial man.

Here then are the rudiments of his tale.

Dad grew up on a farm in a small town in South Africa. His father, who had wanted to be a lawyer, was sworn by his own dying father to take over running the family's small-town hotel. It was a painful oath, borne stoically by my grandfather, but bitterly resented by his wife. The couple had three sons. The eldest was their mother's favorite; the youngest, my football hero namesake, their father's favorite; my father, nobody's favorite.

Because there was no proper school in the small town, my father was sent to the nearest big town, which had a boarding school structured in the strict British tradition, including the routine hazing of new boys. It was a frightening experience. My father told me about one event in this hazing in which the older boys, borrowing from a scene in

Shakespeare's *King Lear*, blindfolded the initiates and confused them by leading them up and down stairs until they believed they were high up on a roof. Then they made the young boys jump blindfolded from the "roof," which was actually just one or two steps off the ground. The boys experienced terror at the thought of jumping (or being pushed) from a great height, then shock when they hit the ground so soon. Even as he told the story, I could see my father eyes narrow as he reexperienced the trauma. He would have been seven or eight at the time.

When Dad was nine years old, something terrible happened to him at school. Nobody knows what it was, but in the middle of the night, he rode home from school on his bicycle, a distance of thirty miles. This midnight ride had a fortunate outcome. Recognizing my father's profound unhappiness in boarding school, his parents were able to secure him lodgings with a very kind family in the city, and he became much less unhappy. As an adult, Dad always inveighed against anyone sending their small children to boarding school, and went out of his way to dissuade others from doing so.

In high school my father was skipped a year, so that he was always the youngest and shortest boy in his class—a lowly status that recapitulated his experience as the least-favored son. His years at university and law school are terra incognita as far as I'm concerned. All I remember him saying about them is that law school officials hurried his class through graduation because the world was gearing up for war. They wanted the young lawyers to be eligible to enter the South African army as officers.

My father enrolled in the army and was assigned to the intelligence corps, whose responsibility it was to crack enemy codes. He traveled north through Africa and, toward the end of the war, into Italy. I was certain that Dad's six years in the army must have yielded many interesting stories, but either I was wrong or he simply didn't want to talk about them. Many veterans returning from war avoid talking about their experiences, so I got fragments like:

The men sat around bored, watching two scorpions in a bottle fight to the death.

And:

I was told to tend bar, which I hated. One day the guys trashed the bar, so I complained to the officer in command. He liked me, so he relieved me of that tedious duty.

And:

Jimmy [his best friend] had sex with so many women that he got VD and the Egyptian doctor had to insert a catheter. To warn Jimmy that the catheter would hurt, the doctor said, "Him bite!"

My father and Jimmy laughed at that quaint phrase for years afterward.

THESE TRIVIAL AND HUMOROUS STORIES concealed the sad reality of what really happened to my father during the war. In those years, he lost most of his family. First, his mother died of a burst appendix. Then his younger brother, Norman, was killed in a tank battle. Dad returned home to his bereft father, who recalled how as a child, Norman had developed an abscess in his leg that almost required amputation. "I wish they *had* amputated his leg," the grieving father said. "Then he would still be with us. I'm just glad his mother didn't live to see this day."

Dad's father did not live long after that. He died of a heart attack on the tennis court at age fifty-four, but everyone said he died of a broken heart, mourning his wife and son.

Dad told me about the day he returned to close up the family farm.

"It was raining heavily that day," he said. "It was as though the heavens themselves had opened up and were weeping."

For some time after that, Dad would have frequent nightmares, from which he would wake in a cold sweat, his heart pounding. Initially, he would dream that his family was all back together again—how blissful that must have been!—until a cold, wrenching realization would jolt him awake, time and again, to face the fact that his parents and brother were irretrievably lost. Such nightmares are, of course, classic symptoms of post-traumatic stress disorder.

Shortly after the war, Dad met and married my mother. She was a gracious woman with a steely temperament and a formidable intellect. He adored her; she stabilized him. I once asked my mother whether one loved people despite their faults. "No," she replied. "You love them because of their faults."

Shortly after my parents' marriage I was born, and, two years later, my twin sisters. My mother hemorrhaged badly after their birth, and I've been told she would have died had the midwife not sat by her side all night long, manually clamping down her uterus until the bleeding stopped. So my father almost sustained another grievous loss.

I don't believe my father ever recovered from this series of blows. Although the exuberant elements in his fabric sustained him for a while, he was finally brought down by some combination of his genetic legacy (others in his family had suffered mood disorders) and the traumas of his life, which he struggled to avoid thinking about or dealing with.

His favorite lines from Shakespeare were those spoken by Macbeth after the death of his queen: "She should have died hereafter; There would have been a time for such a word," along with the rest of the famous soliloquy. It was as though Dad were saying, "Of course I know everyone has to die, but why did it all have to happen so soon?"

As I wrote this chapter, I felt a great sadness, realizing all over again how trauma gets passed down from one generation to the next. I think back to Oscar Wilde's quote at the top of this chapter: First we love our parents; then we judge them; and sometimes we forgive them. But if we are lucky, I would like to add, we come to understand them, and with that last step, in the maturity of adulthood, we recapture some of the love we had for them so many years before.

> *Understanding is a key to love.*

Chapter 16

Mysteries of Mood

Midway in the journey of our life I found myself in
a dark wood, for the straight way was lost.

—DANTE ALIGHIERI

We see the world not as it is, but as we are.

—ANAÏS NIN

I remember distinctly the first time I realized that what I did could change my mood. In many ways, it was an unremarkable morning in downtown Johannesburg, long ago. I was in my teens, and for no apparent reason, a gloomy mood had settled in like dark clouds spoiling a fine day. On an impulse I bought an apple and a copy of *MAD* magazine, then caught the bus for home. As the bus meandered along its familiar route, I started to munch on the apple and read the magazine—and before very long, I felt much better. I cannot say why. Maybe it was the tart-sweet taste of the apple, the sugar itself, the magazine's irreverent cartoons, or the view of the well-tended suburban gardens from the upper deck of the bus. By the time I got home, I was in excellent spirits, not the least because I had discovered something new: that I could alter my mood simply by altering my behavior.

Some years later, shortly after my marriage, I discovered that my mood could be modified just as easily in the opposite direction. I had taken to practicing yoga every Sunday morning, but was troubled by reflux that occurred during the upside-down poses. I was prescribed a drug called metoclopramide (which is still on the market as of the time of writing). I took one of the pills, and over the next few hours, I felt a growing sense of gloom. The world seemed empty, the future bleak.

I recognized this feeling as completely out of line with the realities of my life. Newly wed, I was, in general, happier than I could ever remember being. So I suspected that this sudden sadness was an effect of the drug. But how could I be sure? And if it *was* the drug, I wondered, how long would the effects last? At the thought of being stuck in that horrible mental state, I actually burst into tears. Fortunately, the gloom lifted, and within a few hours I was myself again.

It was partly the scientist in me, partly the wish not to throw away something that might help, that induced me to try the drug again. It was the following Sunday, once again before yoga class. This time I was waiting for my mood to drop, and sure enough, it did. I felt a slowing down, fogginess, and emptiness, but this time no gloom. I told myself it was the drug, and that it would pass. I canceled yoga and slept it off.

From that experience I learned several things: first, that chemicals can cause depression; second, that individuals can be specifically susceptible to a particular type of chemical; third, that depression can pass; and finally, that if you know a mood or some other bad feeling is chemical and will pass, then the exact same chemical has less power to bring you down. All these lessons were to stand me in good stead in my career.

Incidentally, I strongly encourage others to look for patterns in what brings you down or makes you feel bad, because that will often suggest a simple and effective strategy—avoidance. One friend of mine, for example, has identified an allergy to the gluten contained in wheat.

She makes a point of discussing it with the waiter whenever we have lunch together, and is thereby able to avoid gluten and enjoy lunch with no unpleasant aftereffects. My friend Tom and I are both allergic to wood mold. I remember one time walking into a restaurant for lunch and soon realizing we'd be ill if we stayed for the meal. Our wives were good-natured about it when we both declared we needed to switch restaurants.

There are all sorts of things that bring people down, one way or another: toxic chemicals, toxic people, places that are too dark or too hot or contain too many cats. I am by no means saying that everyone should avoid people, places, and things that are less than perfect. That's neither feasible nor the formula for a full life. Rather, I am saying that many people are especially sensitive to one thing or another—things that make them feel really ill, physically or mentally. Where possible, it is valuable to identify those triggers and avoid them.

Of course, many people are perturbed by none of the above. If you are one of them, count yourself lucky. My mother was like that, so, as a young person, she thought that more sensitive people were simply making a fuss about nothing. Mom also had the good fortune never to experience a day of depression in her life. As she matured, however, she came to realize how lucky she was to have such a robust constitution, and she became much more empathic toward those who didn't.

And there were many in my family, on my father's side, who suffered from problems with mood regulation, leading me to conclude that depression must run in the family. Indeed, I could virtually track the genes, either from knowing the people or hearing stories about them. My father, as I have described, was a moody man.

His mother I never knew, but I gather she was perennially disgruntled (though it was the general opinion that being stuck in the country gave her much to be disgruntled about), while her sister (my father's aunt) was a picture of melancholia. When my family would come to visit, we'd usually find her in an armchair or in bed, wearing an expression of inconsolable gloom. Later in life she cheered up a good deal.

Being a medical student, I wondered whether some physician might have started her on one of the newly available antidepressants. In any event, I then caught glimpses of the charming and vivacious woman she must have been before she became depressed. And there were several others in my father's maternal line who also suffered from depression and anxiety (which tend to run together in families).

Then there was the good childhood friend of mine Philip, who showed mood swings even in second grade. A very energetic boy, Philip was always breaking rules and getting into trouble, but he also seemed to have a great deal more fun than I had by sticking to the rules. At the same time, Philip could also be moved to tears by tiny setbacks—like not winning a contest in class. Tragically, as an adult, my friend developed full-blown bipolar disorder and ended up committing suicide.

Given this history, it is no coincidence that I have spent a great deal of my professional life treating people with mood disorders and researching the subject. My own personal experiences, along with seeing friends and family suffer, instilled in me a decades-long fascination with the mysteries of mood and a driving need to find novel ways to treat its disorders.

We live in promising times for anyone interested in genetic disorders, and the genetic underpinnings of mood disorders are well established. There is every reason to hope that as we develop better ways to modify the human genome, we will be able to use this technology to treat people with mood disorders. The bad news is that so far, very few people with *any* medical condition have been treated successfully by genetic modification.

What is to be done in the meanwhile? Besides treating patients with available and approved medications and techniques, I have always been drawn to novel approaches that are ready for use right now. Later in this book, I will discuss my role in describing seasonal affective disorder (SAD) and helping to develop light therapy as a treatment for this and other conditions (see chapter 28). Likewise, I will tell you more about my interest in Transcendental Meditation (TM) as a potential treatment for mood disorders and other conditions (see chapter 40). What I'd like to do here is to tell you about two other offbeat treatments for depression that have been a focus of my interest: St. John's wort and Botox.

My interest in St. John's wort was a voyage of discovery. This flowering herb has been reputed to have antidepressant properties for at least three hundred and fifty years. Modern research studies appeared to support these historical claims, and one of my patients, a pharmacist, told me he no longer needed my help since starting himself on the herb. I simply had to investigate!

Imagine my excitement when I discovered, hidden in the bowels of the National Library of Medicine, a three-hundred-and-fifty-year-old German manuscript written by the chemist Angelo Sala. Sala describes an ingenious recipe for extracting the active ingredients from the leaves and petals of the St. John's wort flower with brandy, then using a steel helmet to shelter the elixir from sunlight (which can degrade the active ingredients). Here is a translation of what Sala has to say about the herb.

> St. John's wort has a curious, excellent reputation for the treatment of illnesses of the imagination, which are known by some as phantasmata and by others as mad spirits, and for the treatment of melancholia, anxiety and disturbances of understanding, which sometimes affect highly intelligent people whose primary personality is not melancholic.

And how did Sala assess its potency in comparison to other "cures"? Sala's answer:

> Without overstating the herb's benefits, I effected cures which you can achieve neither with all the rest of your Apothecary nor with the best prescriptions made out of gold, silver, coral, pearls, stone or jewels (even those that have been found to be useful

and wonderful in the treatment of other illnesses). I could not
have treated these patients more effectively. I recognize, even as
I am describing these cures, that novices who have never had
such experiences would be scornful of these claims.

I agree with Sala (though I haven't tried gold, silver, or coral). Based on
both research studies and clinical experience, St. John's wort works,
especially for mild or moderate (as opposed to severe) levels of depression. Several of my patients have used it to good effect for years.

All this exciting old (but rediscovered) information formed the
basis of my book *St. John's Wort: The Herbal Way to Feeling Good.*

One caveat: Like all effective treatments, St. John's wort has side
effects, including sensitizing the skin and possibly the eyes to bright
light; it can also interfere with the levels of other drugs a person may be
taking. It's always a good idea to consult with your doctor before taking
this—or any other—active substance.

The Botox story is my most recent foray into alternative care for
depression. My friend and colleague Eric Finzi is a dermatologist in the
Washington, D.C., area, a researcher and artist who had become fascinated with the emotional impact of one's facial expressions. We all
know that our emotions influence our facial expressions: Feel sad →
look sad. Could the reverse also be true? It's an old idea, one that
Charles Darwin had suggested.

Psychologist William James followed up on Darwin's observation
and speculated that we do not cry because we are sad. We are sad because we cry. Finzi traced the hundred-and-forty-year research trail on
this so-called "facial feedback hypothesis" and reached an inescapable
conclusion: Our facial expressions do affect the way we feel. Frowning
makes people feel bad; smiling makes them feel better. He has beautifully explored this topic in his book *The Face of Emotion: How Botox Affects
Our Moods and Relationships.*

I had long been aware of the substantial research on the facial-
feedback hypothesis and was persuaded of its importance. Following

the recommendation of the Buddhist monk and poet Thich Nhat Hanh, I often assume "the half smile of the Buddha" as I go about my chores (especially the tedious ones), and I find them less unpleasant when I do.

Finzi's observations have particular relevance to people with depression, who often show characteristic (and sometimes fixed) facial expressions. Specifically, the muscles between the eyebrows, the corrugator muscles, which produce vertical frown lines, are overactive in many depressed (and distressed) people. Severely depressed people even develop the "omega sign," so called because the two frown lines between the eyebrows join at the upper end, creating a tentlike shape that looks like the last letter of the Greek alphabet. Finzi hypothesized that these scrunched-up muscles might be sending distress signals back to the brain, thereby aggravating and perpetuating feelings of depression.

As a dermatologist, Finzi had a logical way to test his hypothesis: Botox, more formally known as botulinum toxin, powerfully inhibits muscle contractions. Could Botox help depressed people, Finzi wondered, if it were injected into the corrugator muscles? In a pilot study, he tested the idea in ten of his dermatology patients who were also depressed and was confident he saw a beneficial effect. Finzi was aware, however, as are all depression researchers, that the placebo effect can be powerful—especially when the researcher is as eager as the patient to see improvement.

Clearly a controlled study of Botox for depression was necessary, and that's where I entered the picture. I was at the time running a private clinical research facility, where we had studied many different interventions for depression—mostly pharmaceutical, but also complementary, including light therapy and TM. After talking to Finzi, I was quickly persuaded that his Botox idea was perfect for me and my organization—novel, outside-the-box, ready-to-go, and potentially of great value to people suffering from depression.

In a state-of-the-art clinical trial (random assignment and double-blind control), we tested Botox versus placebo injections into the corrugator muscles of seventy-four depressed people. Before breaking the blind, none of us had any idea what the study would show. In fact, my colleagues on the front lines told me they were quite concerned that so many people were getting better. Could injections between the eyebrows be causing a huge placebo effect? But when we broke the blind, the results were clear. Botox knocked placebo out of the ballpark. Although these are early days for recommending Botox to relieve emotional suffering, I am confident that we have here yet another wonderful weapon against a formidable foe—depression. I am excited to see how this line of research develops, as it may also help others, including people with anxiety or PTSD.

Light therapy, St. John's wort, TM, Botox: What a great adventure it has been to explore such novel ways to help people who suffer the torments of mood disorders. I trace my intense drive and curiosity to explore these avenues to my personal experiences with mood shifts— both pleasant and nasty. My own adversity in this regard has fortunately been small, but I have witnessed exquisite pain in others whom I have loved. Watching people get better—or not—has sustained my quest to understand the mysteries of mood, and to pursue new and effective treatment for mood disorders that can be so devastating.

You carry a great laboratory in your own mind. If you use that laboratory, by a careful process of observation, you will discover wonders within yourself and may find solutions to the great issues that confront you (and others)—including how best to regulate your sense of well-being.

Chapter 17

Medical School

If you want to go fast, go alone.
If you want to go far, go together.
—OLD AFRICAN PROVERB

In South Africa, still using the British system, high school graduates wishing to study medicine go straight to medical school—unlike their U.S. counterparts, most of whom do a four-year undergraduate degree first. Under the South African system, we studied premed subjects for three years, followed by three clinical years.

In the preclinical years, our lecturers loaded us up with huge volumes of material, more than I had ever encountered in my entire life. I was blessed with a good memory but cursed with a poor attention span, especially for volumes of boring stuff. My options were simple: Either I would do badly, or I would have to find a way to do well.

My yoga teacher at the time had a favorite saying: "If you need a helping hand, look at the end of your right arm." But the hand at the end of my right arm did not want to turn the many pages of the many textbooks we were assigned. Instead, it wanted to turn on the radio or pick up a work of fiction or poetry or open the fridge to inspect its contents (just a reconnaissance mission, of course).

Clearly, self-help had reached its limits. Luckily, there was a solution from elsewhere: two great friends, whom I credit with getting me through medical school well. Ken Polonsky and I had been best friends in high school and had frequently studied together. In medical school, we became dissection and lab partners, and continued to study together. Ken was a brilliant student, and far better than I at sticking with a text. To my many suggestions that it was time for a break, he would respond patiently, "Let's just do another few pages and then we can take a break." So, miraculously, all the studying got done—and enjoyably so.

After a few years, we met another medical student, Wil Lieberthal, who succeeded in getting an A in virtually every subject at medical school. Wil generously shared with us his methods for taking notes and organizing information, which made us more effective. So we became a trio, sharing notes and information, and helping one another cover far more territory than would have been possible for any one of us alone.

When I recently asked Wil how he thought we all benefited from working together, he replied—with this book in mind—that our collaboration was a good example of the gift of adversity. At medical school, he explained, the demands were overwhelming. We were drowning in a huge volume of information that we were expected not only to memorize, but to absorb and integrate. It was too much for any individual to do with a high level of excellence. The key to our collaboration was our triumvirate. As to how it worked, Wil says:

> We liked each other and trusted each other. Working together made the whole thing seem like fun. There's no point asking, "What did each of us contribute?" though I'm sure we all had our own skills that we brought to the problems at hand. We had the benefit of three good brains, working together to figure things out and share information. We were driven to succeed, and all had the same goal—to achieve excellence. It was an

amazing collaboration from which we all benefited. The sum was greater than its parts. We talked constantly and supported one another through a difficult and stressful program. We all wanted to do well, and enjoyed each other's success. We managed to subordinate our competitive instincts for the general good. For me, the take-home lesson is that you are better off collaborating than competing.

I am confident that without Ken and Wil, my medical school performance would have been mediocre. As it was, all three of us graduated with high honors. On the basis of these results, I was admitted into a first-rate U.S. psychiatric residency without an interview, which would certainly not otherwise have happened. Ken went on to a distinguished career as an endocrinologist and is, at the time of writing, dean of medicine at the University of Chicago. He and his wife, Lydia, remain close friends of mine to this day. Wil went on to become a distinguished researcher and nephrologist. (As a side benefit of our collaboration, he also married my sister.)

This medical school experience taught me the power of collaboration, a crucial skill for everyone. I realized that people have complementary skills, and that usually one person can't do the job as well alone. As Wil said, it was much more fun working together, and I remember joking, laughing, and sharing ideas on many occasions. In fact, more than any specific thing I learned in class, the lab, or the wards, learning how to collaborate was to give me the biggest payoff in the years to come. This lesson stood me in good stead as a researcher, where collaboration with others is crucial. Likewise in the clinical trials business, where as CEO I needed to know not only how to collaborate but how to foster collaboration in others. Finally, as a psychiatrist and coach, I help people who have to function in groups in order to achieve their goals. Having successfully done so myself in different settings enables me to help others in this regard.

One other point worth mentioning about medical school is that it afforded me firsthand exposure to the extreme contrast between the clinical care provided to whites versus blacks. The Johannesburg General Hospital, which at that time was exclusively available to whites, was a showpiece of high-quality care, equivalent to the best London hospitals of the day. Baragwanath Hospital, located beside the black township of Soweto, presented a radically different picture. I could go through the differences point by point, but suffice it to say that the one was clean and shining, with plentiful supplies and beds spaced a good distance apart; the other was dirty and crowded. On one occasion, I actually saw a rat running across the hospital floor.

The other great difference between the hospitals lay in the degree of pathology they housed, which was due to several factors: Blacks were poor, lacked education, and received little primary care. As a consequence, at Baragwanath, the patients were much sicker, and their prospects for recovery far bleaker. It was heartbreaking to see so many daily tragedies of people who could have been saved if only . . . if only they had understood the gravity of their situation, if only they had been able to take a few days off to get the problem sorted out sooner.

Sadly, even in the United States we see a comparable (though less extreme) discrepancy between the care available to the rich versus the poor. Maybe improved collaboration between different interested parties (for example, the for-profit and nonprofit sectors) will offer a better solution to this ancient and ubiquitous problem.

> *Success in life depends, to a large extent, on your ability to collaborate. Although the ability to work alone is a virtue, interdependence is increasingly necessary in our complex world.*

Chapter 18

A Brush with the South African Police

Give me that man
That is not passion's slave, and I will wear him
In my heart's core.

—SHAKESPEARE, *HAMLET*

On returning from a long trip to Europe, I was happy to see the girl I had been dating, as she was to see me. At the end of the evening, we encountered a familiar problem—where to go to spend some private time.

To give you a context, I should explain that in Johannesburg in the 1960s and 1970s, college and graduate students generally lived with their parents. Also, it was not commonly accepted (at least not in my home) that you bring your date home, go into the bedroom, shut the door, and emerge whenever. So my girlfriend and I had a problem, which we solved by parking near a lake. We'd never been disturbed before—until now.

On arriving at "our" spot, I could tell right away by the light of the moon that some change was in the works. Wooden poles had been installed in such a way as to make the area unwelcoming—the parking lot had pretty much disappeared. But we'd been apart for weeks, so, undeterred, we settled down to spend some time together.

It should have come as no surprise when a police car drove up. A cop with a flashlight climbed out and started asking questions in Afrikaans. What were we doing here? Didn't we realize that this place was being turned into a rose garden for "*oordentelike mense*," decent people? he sneered. Fortunately we were both fully clothed, except I had no socks on. One had gone missing earlier, as socks tend to do, so I had decided to leave the other sock off as well.

The police demanded that we follow them to a police station; I countered by insisting that my father, who was my lawyer, be contacted. I didn't trust what might happen to us if we went to the police station alone. Only a few years earlier, my cousin John had been locked in solitary confinement and tortured for months by the South African police. (I will tell you more about him in chapter 45.) So I was understandably terrified of being thrown into God knows where—a dungeon? a black hole? a gulag? They refused to contact anyone and said they would go looking elsewhere until I had changed my mind.

I took the bait. As they drove around the lake, I seized the opportunity to drive to my girlfriend's home, not far away. Of course, they followed in hot pursuit. I jumped out of the car to run into her house. A policeman grabbed my arm. I threatened to sue him if any harm came to me.

As I write this account, I realize that at that time in South African history, before the Soweto riots had changed everything, the police must still have believed they were accountable and had to obey certain rules. I gather that such niceties fell by the wayside in the years that followed. Also, though I didn't know it at the time, in their eyes I was only a minor scofflaw. They kept their special treatment for people they regarded as political threats.

In the end, the police allowed me to enter my girlfriend's home and phone my father, who arrived shortly. I was proud (and relieved) to see "the Fixer" swing into action, sweet-talking the policemen in Afrikaans, making my girlfriend's parents feel at home (though in fact it *was* their home), reassuring my girlfriend and myself. He called me aside and said, "The one policeman is slurring his words. If he gives us any trouble, we'll demand that he take a Breathalyzer test." The Fixer's magic worked. Everyone settled down. We agreed that we would all go to the police station to file a report. No charges would be filed.

As I drove to the station, the police flagged me over to the scene of the crime with a flashlight. I obeyed and stopped the car. My girlfriend, her parents, my father, and the policemen had driven ahead and were all gathered at the scene. "Step out of the car," said one of the policemen. I obeyed. He held up something that unfortunately looked very much like my missing sock. "Is this yours?" he said. "Lift up your trouser pants." I did so. I will not soon forget the sight of my pale ankles illuminated by the moon—the cynosure of all eyes. Nobody said anything; there was nothing to say.

That was the high point. The rest was anticlimax—a routine visit to the police station, a perfunctory good night to my girlfriend, then back home to my parents, my sisters, and my grandmother. The old lady pretended naïveté about the whole matter and had the last word, as she often did: "I'm just glad you didn't fall into the lake," she said.

CLINICIANS HAVE LONG RECOGNIZED hot and cold states, states of high and low arousal respectively. In states of high arousal, such as sexual desire, anger, or exuberance, we tend to be "passion's slaves" and act rashly. One aspect of wisdom is to learn to tame your passions.

Self-knowledge helps—to understand one's triggers, specific things that are likely to set you off. So does good self-care, such as handling stress; getting enough sleep, exercise, and rest; and eating regularly. To these last two points, a 2011 study by Shai Danziger (and colleagues at the Ben-Gurion University of the Negev in Israel) showed that the likelihood of a prisoner receiving parole was directly related to whether the judge had just eaten and how many cases he or she had already seen that session. The better fed and rested the judge, the more likely the prisoner was to be paroled. One practice that has helped many people (myself included) feel calm and centered, and therefore to keep a cooler head and to make better decisions, is meditation, which I discuss further in chapter 40.

Perhaps some of you also have memories of moonlit nights when you were passion's slaves. If so, I hope you all got home as safely as I did that evening.

> *Tame your passions before making important decisions; good judgment is most likely to occur when the head is cool, the body is rested, and the stomach is full.*

Chapter 19

A Brutal Attack

You only live twice: Once when you are born and
once when you look death in the face.

—IAN FLEMING

It was another evening on the town in Johannesburg—same car, different girl. We'd had a pleasant Chinese dinner with friends and I was driving her home. It was early yet, so we decided to park for a while in a shadowy lane in her neighborhood. The night was warm and dry, and the car was filled with the fragrance of my girlfriend's perfume— Impulse, it was called. In those days, Johannesburg was not yet the violent city it has since become. The suburban street was quiet and seemed peaceful. It felt like a perfect time simply to visit and chat. I was an intern now, with a room in the doctors' residence. Trysts in cars were fortunately a thing of the past.

We chatted about such bygone times. Had I ever been busted by the police in a parked car? she asked. I told her my story. She told me hers— an innocent adventure with a smooth-talking Italian on a hilltop, high above the lights of Rome. At that moment a voice came through the window on my side of the car (we drove on the left-hand side of the road in South Africa, which meant the driver's seat was on the right): "Yes," said the voice.

Oh, no, I think to myself, *not the cops again, but at least I am fully clothed.* At that moment a rock comes crashing through the windshield. This is not the cops! We are under attack. The smell of dust and pine trees mingles with the sensation of powdered glass in my nostrils. The window on my side of the car is also shattered, and I feel a sharp object coming at me again and again. I grab the assailant's hand with my right hand and grind it against the broken glass of the window. With the other hand I honk the horn; my girlfriend screams. The noise activates the neighborhood; lights turn on; and the two thugs escape into the darkness.

I throw the car into reverse, spin it around, gun the engine, and drive the half mile to my girlfriend's home. As she helps me up the front steps, the same question occurs to us both: "Are you hurt?" She says she is fine; I am less sure. The warm liquid running down my side feels suspiciously like blood, yet I feel no pain, just a vague faintness, and I'm wobbling on my feet. The wobbliness is accompanied by a strong resolve to get where I need to go, which lets up only when I reach the living room, where my legs give way and I collapse on the carpet in a pool of blood.

My girlfriend and her parents hustle me into their car, and soon we are en route to the hospital. As I breathe in and out, I feel sharp pains in my chest with each breath. I know this means that my chest cavity has been pierced and my lung on that side has collapsed. I am surprisingly calm and free of pain (later I realize that, as part of the acute stress response, endorphins pour into the bloodstream). I think to myself, *If I die, it will be okay.* But I get to the hospital in time and they lay me down on a gurney, get an IV running, and prep me for surgery. My friend Wil, a fellow intern at Johannesburg General, has been called and is standing beside me. Just as they are about to wheel me into the operating room, I am suddenly overwhelmed by the worst pain I have ever felt in my life. "Get me under!" I scream. "Get me under!" And they do.

I had requested the surgeon for whom I would subsequently do my surgical internship. It was April first, and when they called to tell him that his future intern had been stabbed, he thought someone was playing an April Fools' joke on him. Yet he came promptly and did a good job. I was in the ICU at first, then a private ward. The surgeon came to visit and described my injuries; I had been stabbed several times with a sharp instrument through multiple organs. "They missed your aorta by about this much," he said, holding his thumb and forefinger close together. "One quarter of an inch the other way and you would have been gone." As I have told this story to others, many relate to it and tell me how they too have missed death by about a quarter of an inch. It seems that life is more precarious than we like to think.

The surgery was successful, and the short-term recovery standard—I was young and in good hands—but aftershocks from the attack would come back to haunt me years later. The staff was very kind, and friends visited. The professor of surgery asked whether I had not been persuaded by the amazing outcome of the operation to become a surgeon. No, I said, psychiatry was where my interest lay.

Dr. T, my former Latin teacher who was now a good friend, came to visit. "How are you feeling?" she asked. "Stupid," I said. "What an idiot I was to be parked like that in a shady lane." "Ah, Norman," she said in her rich Italian accent, "Parking in shady lanes is part of life. You cannot turn your back on life."

Many years later, on a trip to Naples, I went walking of an evening with a friend along a road atop a hill. Cars were parked alongside the road with newspaper covering their windows. "What's that all about?" I asked. "Ah," he said, "it is the young people. They have nowhere else to go." I understood afresh my Latin teacher's sympathetic philosophy in the aftermath of my attack. But I also realized that it might be fine to park with a lover in a lane in Naples, but Johannesburg, even before the Soweto riots, had already become too dangerous for such adventures.

As I think of the attack today, I am reminded of Aesop's fable about the one-eyed doe. Because she had only one eye, she would always graze on a seaside cliff top, chosen so that she could turn her good eye toward the land to detect hunters before they could shoot her. Instead, she was killed by an arrow shot from a passing ship. Aesop's moral: Danger comes when and where you least expect it. So it was that in my mind, danger to people in cars came from overzealous policemen. Hence, I was unprepared. My mind was anchored on the wrong threat.

Only afterward did I learn about *panga* gangs in Johannesburg, who preyed in pairs on couples parked in cars. Typically, they would kill the man with a *panga* (an African word for a long, sharp weapon), rape and kill the woman, then make off with the car. The police found the men responsible for the attack literally red-handed, in possession of the eighteen-inch sharpened screwdriver they had used to stab me.

Years later, when my son, Josh, was a boy of about nine or ten, he said, "Dad, will you promise me that you will be okay, that nothing bad will happen to you?" I told him I could not promise that, because so many things are out of our control, but that I *could* promise to do every-thing in my power to stay safe. That seemed good enough to reassure him, and I have done my very best to keep that promise. Since I recov-ered from the trauma and acquired a family and other responsibilities, I no longer think, *If I die, it will be okay.* My family needs me—and others need me—and that, more than anything, has made it very important to me to be careful as I move through life.

> *Life is precious but precarious; treat it with the care and respect it deserves.*

Chapter 20

Born Again

Gifts of Survival

But as for me, I am filled with power,
with the spirit of the Lord.

—MICAH, 3:8

I recovered slowly from the incident. When tissues are injured, the body releases chemicals that force you to rest, sleep, and take it easy. When I woke up in the ICU and told the staff I would be out and about in three days, they laughed at me. They were right, of course. I was in the hospital for a week, then convalesced for two weeks more at home. Slowly my strength came back.

I looked at my day planner, so full of tasks to do in the weeks following the accident. I thought, not for the first time, of Robert Burns's comment about how the best-laid schemes of mice and men "gang aft agley." Who did all those tasks? I have no idea. Maybe they didn't get done. As many have said, the cemeteries are full of indispensable people.

As I recovered physically, a new urgency stirred inside me, or rather, it felt as though something entered me from the outside—a force, a power, a drive—that directed me to create, produce, and reproduce. I was like someone swept along in the thrall of a posthypnotic suggestion. My senses were heightened for everything, including a powerful sense of time passing. I had enormous appreciation for being alive. I felt I had to do things with my life—and quickly. I could relate to people who feel as though they have been born again.

Also, I understood how men feel after returning from war: the urge to have a family, to replenish lives lost, and to buttress lives almost lost. In the face of near-death, it was as though my genes were crying out to me to hurry up and reproduce while there was still time.

I met my wife by a curious set of circumstances. So unusual was the attack upon a medical intern that my picture landed on the front page of the paper, along with my father's picture. Leora, who had been a classmate of mine in third grade before transferring to another school, recognized me and remembered me fondly. (She says I had defended her against a class bully who had called her stupid. I told him she wasn't stupid, and that apparently had settled the matter.) Leora's father, in turn, recognized my father as a classmate from the horrible country school I told you about. Leora's brother-in-law was a medical student on the same ward where I was interning. Such were the interlinkages of the Jewish subculture of Johannesburg, which was like a shtetl transferred from Eastern Europe to Southern Africa.

Within a year of my attack, Leora and I had met, fallen in love, married, and conceived Joshua. I have often thought of that line from *Julius Caesar*: "There is a tide in the affairs of men, which taken at the flood, leads on to fortune." Being attacked had released such a tide in me, and I took it at the flood. The near-death experience also gave me a lasting appreciation of each day and the opportunity to enjoy and contribute to what each day brings.

> *There is nothing like looking death in the face to make you realize that every single day is a precious gift—to use and enjoy, and not to squander.*

Chapter 21

Boot Camp and the Kindness of Strangers

No act of kindness, however small, is ever wasted.

—AESOP

Basic training in the South African Defence Force was nasty, brutish, and, at six weeks, mercifully short—though not short enough.

How could it be other than brutish? The men who trained and drilled us were the people charged with maintaining the ruling regime—the apartheid government of Balthazar Johannes Vorster, who had been interned during World War II for his pro-Nazi sympathies.

You may well wonder why I (and many others who opposed the mission of the apartheid government) entered its defense force. Simply put, it was mandatory. Even if you left the country, should you ever return—for example, to visit a sick or dying parent—they could draft you there and then.

At an early assembly of candidate officers (mostly young doctors like myself) on the parade ground, a dominee (or preacher) addressed us in Afrikaans. He droned on, and, as you might expect, I wasn't listening very carefully, until suddenly my ears pricked up: "And those who don't accept our Lord Jesus Christ will be cursed," he said, "and this will be no ordinary curse but *'n ewige vloek*—an eternal curse." *What the heck am I doing here?* I asked myself. *I don't believe in their mission. They think I'm cursed.* Not exactly an ideal relationship. Yet I persevered, and so, I suppose, did they.

The religious question kept surfacing. During a lecture one day, someone entered the room and the lecturer said, "All Jews stand up and file out the back door." Although we had no idea what was going on, we did as we were told. One of the recruits called out, "Watch out when they turn on the showers, guys. It could be gas!" The reality was more benign—a visit from the Jewish chaplain to check up on how we were doing.

One of my tent mates was a tall fellow with dark hair and a perennially grim-faced expression. Because of his looks and ultra gung ho attitude, we called him the Black Knight. He approached me one day and asked whether he could talk to me. I said sure. He asked if I believed in Christ. To keep it simple, I told him I was Jewish and that Jews generally don't believe in Christ. He said, "You seem like such a nice guy. Please consider accepting Christ as your savior. It makes me so sad to think of you burning in hell forever."

I HAD DREADED BOOT CAMP, in part because, having been stabbed only one year before, I felt physically vulnerable. But I looked around at others I knew who had successfully passed through this rite of passage and I said to myself, *If they managed, you'll manage too.* This attitude had worked for me earlier in relation to another rite of passage—my bar mitzvah. The older guys had tried to scare us with stories about how difficult it was to learn the Torah portion that has to be recited publicly—in Hebrew—as part of the ritual. But I looked around and saw that everyone else seemed to have managed, and said to myself, *You'll man-*

age too. Then I set about figuring out how to do so. Strangely, I have used this same line of thought in relation to a far more unpleasant rite of passage—dying. Most of us dread the prospect of dying, including me. But sometimes, when the fear arises, I say to myself, *It's one test that nobody fails. So you'll pass it too.* Accepting death lets you turn your attention to how you can defer the date and make best use of the time you have.

Shortly after we first reached the training ground, the quartermaster issued us each a trunk, which we filled with uniforms and other necessary items. When packed full, the trunk was too heavy for many of us to carry, yet we were told to put it on our head and run to choose our tents. Tents were important, because we all wanted to end up with our buddies. So I lifted the trunk onto my head and started running until, like many other rookies, I went tumbling down with the trunk in my arms and injured my back in the process. That injury was to dog me throughout my year in the army and is a simple example of the stupidity that was everywhere in evidence. The brass knew that many of us couldn't carry the trunks, but risked injuries anyway as part of the hazing. Knowing that many people would fall over, they had positioned troops along the route to the tents. With laughs and hoots, the troops scooped up the trunks and took them to our tents for us.

Luckily, a medical school friend, Ian, had saved a place for me in his tent, which was full of other classmates—a great comfort, since we kept the same tentmates throughout, even when we moved from the base training ground to a campsite in the bush. Our camaraderie was sustaining. We played bridge and told stories—like how the major who headed up the camp would routinely get drunk at night and set off cherry bombs under an overturned bucket, all for the thrill of watching the bucket jump.

OVERALL I MANAGED FINE, though one exercise threatened to further damage my back. The task was to divide into pairs, and take turns carrying each other to and fro across a long field. It was clear that you should pair up with someone close to your own size, which I thought I had done. He carried me easily across the field and deposited me on the other side. It was only then that I took a proper look at my partner's physique, which was that of a bricklayer or farmhand. My back groaned at the mere idea of hoisting him up, let alone lugging him across the field. He read my face in a flash and said, "Never mind, jump back on. They'll never know the difference." So he hauled me back across. I never learned his name; nor did we ever have a conversation before or after. But I am convinced to this day that I owe the health of my back to the kindness of that stranger.

The kindness of strangers: It is hard to think the phrase without thinking of Blanche DuBois, speaking the famous line from *A Streetcar Named Desire* in her rich Southern accent: "I have always depended on the kindness of strangers." Blanche is a tragic but not entirely sympathetic character, and I suspect that few theatergoers identify with her. Nevertheless, there is something poignant about that line, something we can all relate to, because at important times in our lives, most of us have depended, or will depend, on the kindness of strangers.

I perhaps owe my very existence to the kindness of a stranger. When my mother was in the advanced stages of pregnancy with me, she and my father went to a rugby match. After the match was over, there was a stampede to get out of the stadium. My parents got separated in the teeming crowd, the kind of mass movement in which people get trampled, and my mother became alarmed. Just then, a big, burly man moved her against a wall and formed a cage around her with his arms and back, so that the crowd would move around him and not crush her (and me).

In the past several years, since I have begun to meditate regularly, I am convinced that strangers are kinder to me than before. For example, one rush hour I got a flat tire and was standing at the side of the highway, waiting for AAA to arrive. Within a few minutes, Fritz, a middle-aged gentleman in a Town Car, stopped to help me replace the tire (actually, he did it while I watched). He even escorted me to a nearby tire place, because my spare was in bad shape. Fritz refused to take any money, but did give me his business card: It turned out that he owns a limo business. I have called upon his professional services many times, and he has become a friend. I also let the neighborhood Listserv know about this Good Samaritan, and he has received a great deal of new business from them as well. It feels good to be able to return a favor.

In such a way, the kindness of a stranger, especially when it is needed most, can ripple across society. I suspect that I receive more kindness since beginning to meditate because I *feel* more kindness toward others, and it probably shows.

AT BOOT CAMP, then, I had learned for myself the lesson that Aesop taught thousands of years ago in his tale about the lion and the mouse. As you may recall, the lion spares the mouse's life, and the mouse promises to repay the kindness someday. The lion is amused: "What could a little mouse like you do for me, the King of the Jungle?" But sometime later the lion gets caught in a hunter's net and the mouse indeed comes to his rescue, and gnaws through the net to set the lion free. The moral of the fable holds that no act of kindness, however small, is ever wasted.

> *In contemplating a difficult path, remember that many others have gone that way before you. If they could succeed, then with a little hope, resourcefulness, and help from others, the chances are that you can too.*

Chapter 22

Homeland

Two Views of Sickness and Healing

A wise man proportions his belief to the evidence.

—DAVID HUME

had never even heard of the "homeland" of Bophuthatswana before I was sent there after boot camp. Under apartheid, the theory was that black South Africans would be given their own "homelands," while white South Africans would stay in *their* part of the country. Even at the time the idea seemed ridiculous, as indeed it turned out to be: about 80 percent of the population, the blacks, were to be squeezed into about 17 percent of the land—and by no means the best land. The "homelands" were a patchwork quilt of tracts, often disconnected from one another, that included no cities, ports, or mineral-rich lands. Bophuthatswana was one of these homelands.

The government had decided that some of the military doctors would provide medical care for the homelands, which were severely underserved. The doctors were to work in military uniform so that the residents would regard the army as a benevolent presence. I was one of these doctors, lucky to be serving my time in a setting so much more interesting than a military base. Also, the homeland was not far from my own home in Johannesburg, where Leora was by now in the final month of pregnancy. Telephone service between the homeland and Johannesburg was poor, which was a blessing in a way, as the long letters I wrote her have sharpened my memory of the place.

The George Stegman Hospital consisted of a sprawling collection of buildings, most of them prefab, joined by concrete corridors that were covered by a roof, but open at the sides. The healthier patients sat or lay out on the lawns, sunning themselves in their red-and-white-striped hospital garb, while the sicker ones remained inside in bed. TB was rife; AIDS had not yet arrived (which was just as well, as needles were routinely reused after being soaked in disinfectant). The gardens, beautifully tended, were planted with aloes and flowering annuals. The general feeling of the place was peaceful, cheerful, and exotic. Peacocks strutted around the lawns, providing a final decorative flourish.

The hospital nestled at the foot of a ridge, or *koppie,* on which a cottage had been built for two military doctors. I was the first to arrive and was greeted by two of the hospital staff: the housekeeper, who introduced herself as Tannie (Afrikaans for Auntie), and Dr. R, an intense middle-aged man who ran the hospital, together with his wife. He also led services in the small church just within the gates of the compound. "We are not just interested in the patients' bodies," he said as he showed me around the grounds, "but in their souls as well.

"All the time, we are up against the witch doctors," he continued. "They give the patients their *mutis* [the native word for medicines]. Then, if the patients get better, they take the credit for it. If the patients stay the same, the witch doctor says, 'If you hadn't come to see me when you did, it would have gotten worse.' When they can't help the patients, they say, 'You should have come to see me sooner. Now you'll have to go to the hospital.' If we make the patients better, the witch doctors take the credit for sending them here. If the patients die here, they blame us and say the hospital is a place of death."

In addition to the regular worship service, Dr. R and his wife would often mix faith with their own *mutis*. When a person came in with a seizure disorder, for example, Dr. R's wife, who managed the neurology clinic, would say a prayer to get rid of the seizures, then prescribe an anticonvulsant. If the seizures disappeared, patients had no way of knowing what had made them better. Given the view of disease held by the tribal Tswanas, they were more likely to attribute recovery to the eradication of evil spirits by the power of the white man's prayer than to his tiny pills.

As he showed me around the hospital on that first day, Dr. R introduced me to another fascinating part of the area's history. As district surgeon for the area, he was called in to investigate all suspicious deaths. He told me about a few such incidents, which I shared with Leora—an anthropologist by training—in one of my letters:

Last year [Dr. R had said] we had a case involving twelve witch doctors, who were accused of murdering an old black man for the purpose of obtaining body parts for their mutis. *The corpse—or, rather, what was left of it—was found out in the bush near his home. When I was called in to see it, I found that the right hand had been cut off at the wrist and the left foot at the ankle. All the rest of his bones remained, but all the organs had been removed, and the entire corpse had been skinned except for a small portion of scalp. It was evident that the hand and foot had been cut off while the man was still alive, and that the rest had been removed after he had died. This is typical of a medicine murder, because the parts of the body removed while the person is still alive are believed to be more powerful for making medicines than those parts removed after death.*

The witch doctor usually gives some painkiller, probably more to keep the victim quiet than to alleviate suffering, and then proceeds to cut off the requisite body parts. The right hand and left foot are particularly prized for their presumed potency. The stumps are tied after amputation to prevent the victim from bleeding to death before all the vital portions have been removed.

The twelve accused were brought to trial. The case initially rested on the evidence of an old woman, who saw the dim figures of the murderers and heard the victim's distant cries. Later, one of the witch doctors turned state's evidence to avenge himself on the others, who had held back his fair share of the liver. The witch doctors got a senior advocate from Johannesburg to defend them, and he soon broke down the key witness, the old woman. She could remember neither the day on which the murder had occurred nor the time of night, which is understandable for an old woman living in the bush, far away from clocks and calendars. On the basis of this alone, the case was dismissed, as the judge regarded the evidence of the renegade witch doctor as insufficient grounds on which to pass judgment. The witch doctors were therefore all set free and are still no doubt practicing their arts right here in the community.

Now sometimes an innocent death can look like a medicine murder but may not be one. For example, about three months ago there was a case of some children who went off to play in the long grass. When evening came, they set about herding the sheep and cattle back to the kraal. One little boy was assigned to chase the animals from behind while the others herded them toward the enclosure. The older boys and the cattle returned home by evening, but the smaller boy, who could not see above the tall grass, lost his way. His body was found some days later with the flesh of the right arm and right leg cleared off it. Once again I was called in to examine the body in situ. As I approached the body, a veld rat ran out of the boy's sleeve. Closer examination revealed that all the flesh had been removed by rodents and that there had been no foul play, the boy having died of exposure. Nevertheless, the villagers were unhappy about my opinion. They felt sure that a witch doctor had been at work and set about finding and denouncing the person. They chose some innocent old woman, who is sure to suffer for the "crime." They'll be too scared to kill her, though, because then the white authorities will step in and they will be charged with murder.

. . .

THINGS WERE GETTING curiouser and curiouser, as Alice might have said. By the time Tannie showed me up to the cottage on the *koppie*, I was sun-drenched and dazed by the heat and strangeness of the place. The hillside was dotted with euphorbias, huge candelabra-shaped cactuses. From the terrace on the *koppie*, you could see the large house of the local chieftain, perched on the hillside across from the hospital, as well as the dirt road that led to the little town of Saulsport.

For the next several months I would call the cottage home. My colleague Ivor would join me there, and later so would Leora and our baby son, Josh. At night the peacocks gave off their bloodcurdling cries, and I would lie awake, imagining a person stranded on the koppie, screaming, his right hand severed at the wrist.

There were about four hundred patients in the hospital—far too many to be properly treated by Dr. R and his wife, even with the help of Ivor and myself, who divided up our duties according to our interests. As you can imagine, I gravitated to the psychiatric department, which had both inpatient and outpatient facilities. For "occupational therapy," patients tended to the hospital gardens and made pottery, which was sold. I'm not sure whether they were paid for their services, but I do know that some felt exploited.

The Tswanas believed that illness and other forms of adversity were caused by the evil spirits of the ancestors, brought down upon them by another's ill will or envy. The witch doctor's *muti* worked, therefore, by eradicating the evil spirits. According to one white professor who taught us African medicine, the Western doctor's explanation of illness was much less satisfying to native Africans than the witch doctor's, because the Western doctor explained only *how* an illness arose (such as by infection with germs). The witch doctor answered a more fundamental question: *why* an illness afflicted a particular person.

On one occasion, a young woman was brought to the psychiatric hospital because she heard the evil spirits of the ancestors talking to her. I wasn't sure whether she belonged there. Might not the voices be right in line with cultural beliefs? I asked Joseph, a psychiatric nurse who had become a friend. "Ah, no," he said. "It would be okay if she dreamed about the evil spirits of the ancestors, but she should not be hearing their voices." That taught me a valuable lesson: that I needed to understand the *details* of a person's culture before I could develop an accurate understanding of his or her illness.

At the outpatient clinic, I learned that men who came in complaining of general weakness usually had problems with potency, though custom held that this subject never be directly addressed. In an analogous way, women who complained of general weakness were usually having fertility problems. In either instance, there was nothing specific to be done.

To send all these people away empty-handed, however, would have been heartless. Luckily, a welcome remedy was available—vitamin B_{12} injections. I have no idea whether these injections did anything specific for the people who received them, but they all left very satisfied and grateful. "Injections are where the Western doctor beats the witch doctor," Joseph told me, "because the witch doctor cannot give injections."

No matter what was happening in the hospital, everything stopped for the white staff at eleven a.m. for tea and sandwiches, which were served in the shade of a large tree. At one such gathering, the group discussed how they might acknowledge the work of two missionaries who had spent several months volunteering their time as administrators for the hospital. Someone suggested giving them a useful household item—a casserole dish, perhaps. "Ah, no," said the payroll master, a portly man. "That is very expensive and our funds are so limited. How about a record of gospel songs instead?" Everyone agreed.

Although I was able to go home from time to time, I was often on call in the cottage on the *koppie*. One day, I saw a wasp putting daubs of mud on the corner of an overstuffed chair. She left and returned several times, and I watched as she built her home, before deciding I had better put a stop to it. So I shut the window and saw the wasp bang up against it several times, spattering it with the mud intended for her home (my chair). Eventually she flew away, and I thought that was the end of the story. Then, to my amazement, she came flying in through a window on the opposite side of the house, back to her spot on the chair to keep building her nest. Perhaps because I have always had such a lousy sense of direction, I was deeply impressed that a creature with a brain the size of a pinhead could have such a good sense of her position in space as to find this alternate route into my living room. I realized too that the urge to build a home is not uniquely human.

When Josh was one month old, he and Leora joined me at the cottage, our first home as a family. We were delighted to be there, a family together for the first time. As any couple with a normal infant can attest, the baby casts a spell over the new parents, who regard the little creature as a marvel—which, in fact, it is. But parents of a newborn can also attest that it can be exhausting—especially if the baby wakes often. And indeed, Leora and I were chronically exhausted as a result of both sleep deprivation and the intense heat. The small house on the *koppie* had no air-conditioning, and the African sun beat down upon it all day long.

It was a happy day when a sturdy Tswana woman named Elizabeth presented herself at the door and asked whether she could be of help. She had good references, and Leora and I were both sleep-deprived. It was a no-brainer. We negotiated an agreement with Elizabeth, and I thought all was settled. But the next day Tannie arrived and asked how much we were paying Elizabeth. When we told her, she adopted a sour expression. That would not do, she said. The other maids would complain that they weren't getting as much and we would cause trouble for everybody (meaning the other whites). We nodded our heads respectfully. But once Tannie had left, we told Elizabeth that all would remain as we had agreed, on condition that she said nothing to anybody about her salary. To my knowledge, she never did.

. . .

LEORA AND I remained intrigued by the ritual murders that had taken place in the vicinity. She said they sounded like the famous *muti* murders of Natal, a region of South Africa. Anthropologists theorized that ritual murders typically occurred when the balance of power in a village was disrupted, so that someone saw a need for unusually power-ful medicine to restore social equilibrium. In a 2001 article in the *South African Historical Journal,* historian Rob Turrell elaborates further:

> The ritual killing of a human was required for the acquisition of extraordinary power. And extraordinary power was required to win competitive advantages in chiefly rivalries over people and land. This was why *muti* murders were closely associated with chiefly politics. Still these murders were exceptional in pre-colonial politics and were only committed in the face of an ex-tremely serious challenge to chiefly power.

What disruptions of power might have occurred in Bophuthatswana to provoke the *muti* murders described by Dr. R? One can only speculate. There might, of course, have been competition among the local chief-tains. On the other hand, does it seem too far-fetched to wonder whether the local witch doctors, outflanked by mission hospital doctors with their alternative views of illness, their powerful injections, and their competing theology, might have felt the need to acquire some extraordinary powers of their own?

WHEN WE RECEIVED WORD from the military that our four months at the George Stegman were over, Leora and I left the homeland with regrets. It had been a good time for us. The local people were gentle and surprisingly upbeat despite their poverty, poor nutrition, and illness. They seemed grateful for any help we could give. In that regard, the army's mission had been a success. I felt I had been useful. Thanks to Elizabeth, Leora had been able to rest and recover, and we had both come to love the dreamlike landscape. We had even become accustomed to the peacocks screaming through the night.

The hospital was in the news a few months later when the entire payroll for a month went missing. They caught the thief: It was the portly payroll officer who thought that a casserole dish was too expensive a thank-you gift for the departing missionaries who had volunteered to work at the hospital for many weeks.

Years later I returned to the George Stegman, which remained a working hospital. The basic infrastructure was still in place, but it had not been maintained in its former pristine condition. There were cracks in the buildings and concrete corridors. The beautiful gardens were overgrown with weeds. There were no peaceful patients lying out in the sun, and no peacocks.

This is what I learned from my time in Bophuthatswana:

Faith is a powerful medication.

You can be happy without much in the way of material possessions.

And acceptance of one's lot in life is an important key to happiness.

Chapter 23

Namibia

Confronting Fears

All the world is a very narrow bridge, and the
most important thing is not to fear at all.

—RABBI NACHMAN OF BRATSLAV

April 1976: The plane wended its way through the mountains and
touched down on the runway in Windhoek, the capital of Southwest Africa (formerly German Southwest Africa and now Namibia). I
was to arrive at this new posting ahead of Leora and Josh, with a week
or two to find us a little home before they joined me. In the meanwhile,
I was staying in the officers' quarters, which smelled like a brewery.

The first task for junior medical officers like myself was to examine
the new recruits at Walvis Bay, a dreary seaport on the southwest coast
of Africa. The train ride from Windhoek to the coast, however, was an
unexpected treat—through the Namib Desert, with its golden dunes
and legendary sunsets. Once there, we doctors were dispatched to a
large mess hall, where lines of naked recruits snaked around folding

tables, awaiting their physical examinations. The word "perfunctory" hardly does justice to the procedure, which we referred to by three Afrikaans words—*hande, tande, hoes*—meaning "hands, teeth, cough." The last word was used to check for hernias.

Then came the weekend. The sun was dazzling on the water, and I had friends with cars, who were planning to go fishing and drive to the seaside resort of Swakopmund. The junket was made all the sweeter by schadenfreude: The big brass (majors and colonels) had no private transportation, so they were confined to base, while we lowly lieutenants careened up and down the coast. We caught some fish, had pastries at the famous Café Antoine in Swakopmund, and hung out. I saw a flock of flamingos take flight over a vast lagoon—a cloud of pink feathers in the sky reflected in the water below. I was high on light. In fact, I contracted a mild case of sunstroke, but who cared? I was young, vibrant, and free.

I found an efficiency apartment in a pleasant suburb of Windhoek. The town retained its German character, a remnant of colonial times. A large gingerbread church atop a hill dominated the landscape. Then my family arrived. Leora and I slept on a mattress on the floor, Josh in his crib, and we settled into a peaceful colonial existence. During the day, I worked at the sick bay, where nobody ever seemed to have anything worse than cuts or minor injuries. The staff (nurse and medics) sat around drinking tea and gossiping. Everybody clocked out at five p.m. sharp. Leora and I visited with people to whom we had been introduced by friends in Johannesburg. It was the first time in years that I'd had so little work to do. So we dined in the local restaurants, shopped for the gemstones for which Namibia is famous, and visited friends (with Josh in the backseat—an amiable companion). The Italians have the expression *il dolce farniente*—the sweetness of doing nothing. That is what we enjoyed during our time in Windhoek, and it was sweet indeed.

During one of our social visits, the question of Leora's transportation came up, because she had never learned to drive—a liability in a town that had little by way of public transportation. The truth was that

Leora was terrified of driving, as she confided to our friends. "We have the very person for you," they said. "Mrs. M helped the daughter of some friends of ours, a very timid girl, who thought she would *never* get her license. Yet now she has it. You should contact her."

So Leora did, and lessons began. Mrs. M, who spoke with a thick German accent, knew all the tricks. She trained Leora on the route the examiners invariably took: up the hill, around the gingerbread church, and so on. When the day of the test arrived, however, Leora woke up and said she felt sick. She just couldn't face the test. I had to leave for work, so we decided she would just tell Mrs. M to cancel the test when she arrived. It was difficult to make phone calls from the base, and cell phones, of course, were decades away. So the day ticked by slowly for me as I waited till five o'clock, when I could find out how things had gone. When I arrived home, I was met by a beaming Leora, waving her license at me. "What happened?" I asked. "Well, when Mrs. M arrived, I told her I couldn't do the test. She said to me, 'Vot is ziss nonsense! You vill do ze test! Und you vill pass!' So I did."

We all went out to celebrate.

Mrs. M had understood and demonstrated what many clinicians have come to realize: If someone has a phobia, no amount of analyzing helps. On the contrary: Under the guise of tackling the problem, analysis often fortifies the defenses against corrective action. Instead, you need to encourage (or even push) phobic people into the phobic situation in order to beat it. Leora has driven ever since.

Mrs. M's technique, effective if heavy-handed, resembles a clinical method called flooding, in which the clinician intensively exposes the phobic person to whatever is feared. Although this may work, it is very unpleasant, which is why most clinicians prefer a gentler and equally effective strategy called systematic desensitization. I had occasion to use this latter technique with Joshua after Leora and I had inadvertently traumatized him.

What happened was this: He must have been about two or three years old when, on a visit to South Africa, someone offered to sponsor a course of swimming lessons with a "wonderful" teacher up the road, a local legend who had supposedly saved innumerable children from drowning. That may well have been so, but her technique was radical. As best I could tell, it consisted of throwing the baby into the water and virtually letting him drown before pulling him out. The rationale was that, of necessity, the baby learns to hold his breath, flails around, and willy-nilly becomes waterborne and begins to swim.

We never did reach that goal. Leora and I interceded, though ineffectually at first. "He's screaming!" we protested.

"Better a screaming baby than a screaming mother after the baby has drowned!" shot back the "wonderful" teacher, like an actor who has rehearsed a line too many times.

But she eased up a little, enough so that, to my regret, I brought Josh back for a second lesson. It was as bad as the first, ending with Josh spewing up what seemed like pints of water at the side of the pool. That was it. No more lessons.

Not surprisingly, Josh feared the water for years to come. He wanted nothing to do with it until he was perhaps six or seven, when we joined our local community center. By this time, he was willing to gently explore the possibility of learning to swim.

So we set about our exploration on the steps at the shallow end— first he dipped a toe, then a foot, and so on. Gradually, he became more comfortable with the water until, holding him reassuringly with my arms around his waist, I ventured into the shallow end. And there progress stopped. Josh remained nervous in the water.

The turning point came when a colleague who was a master swimmer saw me and Josh struggling and stopped by to offer advice. "Don't hold him," he said. "Let *him* hold *you*. That way he will have a sense of control, and he will let go of your arm when he feels ready."

That turned out to be sage advice. As my colleague predicted, Josh's confidence grew. Pretty soon he let one hand go, then the other. Once he let go, he would stand on the steps in the shallow end and jump for my arm, at first across short distances, then longer ones. The whole experience felt like a condensed version of the years-long process of letting your child let go of you—and develop independence. Josh went on to become an excellent swimmer and seems to have recovered completely from his early traumatic swim lessons.

TO RETURN BRIEFLY to our stay in Namibia, one last incident is worth relating. In the small town of Keetmanshoop (current population about fifteen thousand), some troops needed their blood drawn. To this end the military dispatched a small plane containing three men: the pilot, the medic (who carried the supplies), and me (who was to draw the blood). After a short ride we touched down at an isolated landing strip (their stand-in for an airport), and walked to the nearest main road to hitch a ride into town.

We were picked up by a pleasant woman in her thirties or forties who was delighted to help out members of the military. "What do you think of all these reports about the terries?" she asked, using the colloquialism for terrorists. She was referring to the South West Africa People's Organization, or SWAPO, an organization of terrorists or freedom fighters (depending on your point of view) that had been operating in Namibia for the previous ten years in what the South African government called the "Border War." In fact, four years earlier, the United Nations General Assembly had recognized SWAPO as "the sole legitimate representative" of Namibia's people. The organization had continued to gain strength and was, at the time of our hitchhiked ride, being supported by foreign aid. So what was I to say? While I wondered—and the medic and pilot remained silent—she drew her own conclusion.

"Well," she said, "as long as we have you boys protecting us, I'm sure we'll be safe." As I thought about my plans to leave for the United States later that year, I realized how easy it is to delude yourself, especially about things that fill you with fear, so that your mind avoids the subject: You really don't want to know. There were signs everywhere that things were reaching a political crisis, but this good-natured woman was disinclined to see it. It would be only a matter of time before SWAPO gained full control of Namibia, where it has been the dominant political party since 1990.

Whether you confront them aggressively or gently, it is important to face your fears. By ignoring them, you increase the risk that trouble will come when you least expect it and are least prepared to deal with it. This lesson applies to governments and organizations as well as to individuals.

Chapter 24

Leaving Home

If you would only recognize that life is hard,
things would be so much easier for you.

—LOUIS D. BRANDEIS

My last military posting was, for the most part, cushy—Natal Command, located in the seaport and vacation resort of Durban. In fact, the base itself was on the seafront, overlooking the Indian Ocean. It was there that I spent most of the remains of my army year, and Leora and Josh were able to join me except for two breaks—when I was sent into the little town of Jozini in Zululand and the small, decrepit city of Ladysmith.

The stint in Zululand was of great value to me: Because there was nothing for the medical officer to do, I lay down on my camp bed for hours at a time, surrounded by lush subtropical greenery, and my back finally had a chance to heal. By contrast, the dreary military base in Ladysmith was a sandy encampment, peppered with poles bearing paranoid slogans, such as "Loose lips sink ships" and "The walls have got ears." The latter statement was made more credible by our prefab lodgings, whose walls were so thin that even a whisper would be clearly audible to an eavesdropper—though I doubt whether there was anything worth overhearing in that outpost. But the poorly insulated walls made the lodgings too cold for a baby, so Leora and Josh returned to Johannesburg.

When I arrived in Ladysmith, the medics seemed unusually pleased to see me. Only later did I learn the reason: The previous doctor had spent long hours looking down the barrel of his gun, as though he were contemplating whether to blow his brains out or not, which had understandably made the medics nervous. I never found out whether he received any help for his problems. Some years later, I heard that he had died young. It was another reminder to me of how much suffering is out there, and how important it is to recognize and treat it promptly.

I was due to be released from the army at the end of June 1976, but because I was expected on the job in New York on July 1, I had saved all my annual leave for the end of my tour, which enabled me to be discharged two weeks early. On June 16, I began the painstaking task of checking out, one department at a time. Every office wanted to make sure that I had returned everything that didn't belong to me—uniforms, weapons, library books—and had left no undischarged obligations.

Now, that very same day, June 16, 1976, was the beginning of the famous Soweto uprising. A mandate had come down that schoolchildren in the black townships must be taught their lessons in Afrikaans, a language they despised because it was associated with apartheid. For these young people, this mandate was the last straw in a growing burden of discriminations and indignities. The Soweto Student Representative Council and other groups had planned a peaceful protest, but riots broke out between protesters and police. Once the police fired shots into the crowd, all hope of a peaceful resolution vanished. By the end of that day, the protests were nationwide and hundreds of people lay dead.

We received regular updates about the spreading riots.

As I continued to check out of the military, the University of Zulu-land, which fell under Natal Command, was said to be in flames. Students in other parts of the country protested in sympathy with the students of Soweto. These protests marked the beginning of the violent rebellion that many of us, myself included, had long predicted. As Gandhi had demonstrated to the British in India, it is impossible for a minority to keep a majority indefinitely suppressed. That lesson was to be repeated time and again throughout Africa. But history shows also that an advantaged group does not readily give up its privilege. People have to fight for their rights, and June 16, 1976, marked a turning point for black South Africans in that fight.

Many South African whites had acted as though their privileged way of life would continue indefinitely. For them, June 16, 1976, marked the beginning of the cracks in their walls of denial. These cracks would deepen over the next fourteen years, until 1990, when Nelson Mandela, a "terrorist" in the eyes of many white South Africans, would be released from his prison on Robben Island and begin to build the new South Africa.

Meanwhile, back at Natal Command, I continued to check myself out. Department by department, each administrator signed some little chit to say that I was in good standing, until, at last, I received my papers of release, signed and sealed—and none too soon. Two hours later, the South African Defense Force canceled all military leave, as of that moment, until the crisis was deemed to have passed.

AS I LEFT NATAL COMMAND, I was too tense to reflect on what I had learned from my time in the South African Defense Force, but in the years that followed, I have often thought about it. I had dreaded the year—the forced separation from family, the rigors of training, being sent off to heaven knew where. (During basic training, one officer threatened to send us to a syphilis clinic on the Angolan border—an active war zone—if we messed up on the parade ground, and I had no reason to believe he was joking.) In short, I anticipated the worst. As you know, however, that was far from the case. I witnessed the unspoiled beauty of Southern Africa. I had a chance to help many people—and learned about them in the process. And, most important, I had precious time with my fledgling family in a world where the workday stopped at five o'clock!

What my army year taught me is to make the best of a situation, even when it looks unpromising. As a young person, the idea of taking a year away from my studies and routines was anathema to me. Now I would recommend it to other young people. Go to a foreign place if you can (even a different part of your own country), not just as a tourist but to engage with the local people in a meaningful way. Learn about their culture and worldview.

How strange to think that a time I feared would bring unmitigated adversity turned out to be one of the most wonderful years of my life.

There is yet another lesson to be gleaned here: Just as some people deny and avoid the things they fear, so others amplify fears, exaggerating the difficulty of what lies ahead. In retrospect, that's what I did with regard to military service.

I remember confiding to Dad one Sunday night how much I was dreading going to school the following day. "That's the Sunday-evening blues," he said. "I used to get it all the time—worrying what Monday will bring. But what I've realized is that once Monday morning arrives, by ten or eleven o'clock, everything is going smoothly, and I can't for the life of me remember what I was so worried about the night before. So now on Sunday evenings, I remind myself that things always feel better on Monday—and I never get the Sunday-evening blues anymore." His lesson—and my year in the military—have stood me in good stead with regard to not "borrowing trouble" and worrying unnecessarily—a piece of wisdom beautifully expressed in the book of Matthew (6:34):

Be therefore not anxious for the morrow: for the morrow will be anxious
 for itself.
Sufficient unto the day is the evil thereof.

I RETURNED HOME from the army with only two weeks in which to
launch our little family for the United States, only to find my father in
terrible physical shape. He had been a longtime denier of physical illness, avoiding doctors whenever possible. He and his best friend, Jimmy
(another lawyer), would consult each other about their medical problems. They seemed to share a belief that if you went to a doctor, he
would "discover" some medical illness that, if left alone, would disappear of its own accord. Instead, the doctor would aggravate the situation with a "cure" that was worse than the disease and might end up
killing you.

Unfortunately, Dad's denial could be sustained for only so long.
Now he had severe chest pain, which any medical student could have
recognized as angina. He vehemently protested my diagnosis, however,
perhaps because his own father had dropped dead of a heart attack in
his mid-fifties. Instead, he attributed his chest pain to his "vagus nerve,"
an anatomical structure he'd probably encountered in the course of a
lawsuit. Was he ill? Of course not. He insisted on coming with me to
shop for clothes for America.

Finally, I prevailed upon him to seek medical help. The doctor diagnosed a probable heart attack and admitted him to the hospital at once.
I bade my father farewell at his bedside, not sure if I would see him
again.

The stress of leaving my country, moving to a land I had never even
visited, and saying good-bye to my father, perhaps for the last time—it
all combined to precipitate a state of continuous hiccups, which lasted
for twenty-four hours. Even with powerful medications I could not stop
hiccuping, so much so that I began to fear I would stand up to answer a
question in my residency class in New York City and hiccup instead of

talking. Yet as soon as the plane took off from Johannesburg Airport, with Leora and Josh at my side, a wave of relief came over me and the hiccups simply vanished. I have never seen, before or since, a more striking demonstration of the mind's great power over the body.

I thought back to my father as he lay propped up in his hospital bed, his face ashen, and I remembered his words: "When you go to America, write about us—because we're a bunch of characters, you know." Then he fixed his shrewd lawyer's gaze upon me and added, "But be sure to put on the cover page, 'All characters in this book are entirely fictitious and any resemblance to persons real or imagined is purely coincidental."

Learn to accept reality. It will improve your life and can make the difference between life and death.

Be careful neither to deny danger (either within your own body or from the world outside) nor to amplify fears, thereby needlessly distressing yourself.

PART II

ADULTHOOD

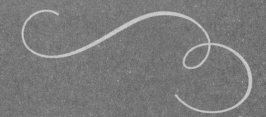

Chapter 25

New York City

A Love Story

Age cannot wither her, nor custom stale
Her infinite variety.

—SHAKESPEARE, *ANTONY AND CLEOPATRA*

f Shakespeare were alive today to wander the streets of New York City—to drop into its restaurants and sample foods from all over the world; to see its wondrous parks, museums, and shows; and to visit its myriad neighborhoods, each with its own special delights—then perhaps he would recall the lines he minted to describe the endlessly fascinating Cleopatra, and apply them to this unique metropolis. I began my own love affair with New York City in the summer of 1976. It was the bicentennial year, when tall ships sailed the Hudson. We visited many parts of the city and settled into the charming neighborhood of Riverdale in the Bronx, which would give me easy access to the New York State Psychiatric Institute, home to the Columbia psychiatric residency.

Our apartment was modest, but it met our needs. The best thing about it was its excellent view of the Bronx from our bedroom window. The worst thing was the landlord, who was notoriously cheap—so much so that the other tenants, who had been there longer than we, were constantly fearful that he would fail to pay the electricity bill. One night, the lights went out in our apartment and either Leora or I said, "It's the damn landlord. He's finally gone and done it." It was the great blackout of 1977.

We took the opportunity to retire early and, in the darkness, slept deeply—until we were woken before daybreak by the phone. It was my mother from South Africa. "How are you doing without light?" she asked. *How does she know the landlord hasn't paid the utility bill?* I wondered. Sensing the confusion in my drowsy silence, she added, "All of New York City is without power." Only then did I look out the window and see the Bronx, usually adazzle, shrouded in darkness.

In this city of strangers, I missed home and family, people who cared whether our lights were working or not, and I was often reminded of that, because when we walked through the neighborhood, we saw older folks who looked very much like the relatives and friends we'd left behind. When they saw us pushing an infant around in a stroller, they responded with emotions, advice, predictions. Once, as we emerged from the elevator, an elderly couple gazed wistfully down at Josh, and the husband said, "So lovely, but before you know it, he'll grow up and go to California and leave you all alone." Another time, we were shopping in Macy's basement and saw an elderly Jewish couple arguing. She was hustling him along, complaining that he was moving too slowly. "Where's the fire, Rachel?" he demanded. "Where's the fire?" The scene could just as easily have played out in a department store in Johannesburg.

It was in that same Macy's basement that I discovered my checks were no good; they were the sampler checks issued by the bank before our personalized checks were ready. In a fury, I made straight for the curiously named Chemical Bank and demanded to see the manager. A sharply dressed young man, Mr. Zara, heard my complaint. "I have money in your bank," I fumed, "and I need to buy things with it, and nobody will accept the checks you issued. What kind of a place is this?"

"You are in New York City now, Dr. Rosenthal," he responded, courteously but firmly. "And as part of living in New York City, this is one of the things you need to deal with." It was such an apt message, so well delivered, that I had no recourse but to accept it. I will never forget Mr. Zara or his name, which is related to the Hebrew word for "stranger," for I was a stranger in a strange land, and I had to accept the ways of that land. A stranger had helped me see that.

Some things about the city were strange in a liberating way. Freedom of expression, for example, like oxygen, is something that is hard to appreciate unless you've gone without it. The first time I became aware of this, I was sitting in a diner with my family, criticizing some politician or policy, when suddenly I had an uncomfortable urge to look over my shoulder and make sure the secret police weren't listening (as might easily have occurred in South Africa). Almost at once I recognized the paranoia of my previous life, still with me. Then it had been adaptive; now it was a vestige of my past. That was the first moment that I was consciously aware of enjoying freedom of speech, and it tasted as sweet as the maple syrup on the hotcakes I was eating.

Curiously, it was my outsider status that led me to my most important observations and experiences in New York City, though I didn't know it at the time. Johannesburg, where I was born and raised, sits at twenty-six degrees south of the equator, whereas New York City is forty degrees north. This means that compared with Johannesburg, the days in New York are much longer in summer and much shorter in winter. I arrived in New York City during the long summer days and felt boundlessly energetic, more than I had ever felt before. I bounced along, not even aware the days were getting shorter, till daylight saving time began in October and clocks were set back an hour. What a difference! All of a sudden, darkness fell before the workday ended. That first day after the time change, as I emerged onto the street, so prematurely dark, a cold wind seemed to blow off the Hudson, and I felt a sense of foreboding. As winter arrived and the darkness deepened, my energy drained away and I could hardly believe I had made so many commitments. Had I been crazy?

I know now that my exuberance, fed by the light of summer, had caused me to overextend myself, so that as the light waned, I had a hard time keeping all those balls in the air. Leora felt the darkness even more than I did. With a baby to look after, she was not able to hibernate, which made life very stressful. Everything improved in the spring, of course, and so it went each year. Through the three years of my residency, we both experienced dramatic cycles of mood and energy in synch with the seasons. Little did I suspect that these cycles, which were so unpleasant for us both, would be a major impetus for my research, or that, just five years after arriving in New York City, I would describe our winter blues as a syndrome and develop a novel treatment for it. Without moving to the north, we would never have experienced the depression of the dark days, nor its unexpected rewards. Once again, adversity was to be a stimulus for creativity and invention.

Look deeply into what makes you different. Understand that difference and develop it, for it may be your greatest contribution.

Chapter 26

Hostile Takeover

The Biological Invasion

"My name is Ozymandias, king of kings:
Look on my works, ye Mighty, and despair!"

—PERCY BYSSHE SHELLEY

When my classmates and I entered the psychiatric residency program at the New York State Psychiatric Institute, part of the Columbia Medical School, we were welcomed by a courtly gentleman named Sid Malitz. Malitz was at that time acting director of the institute, a caretaker position that he was to hold till the arrival of the new director, Ed Sachar.

This was no ordinary changing of the guard, however. The institute had long been a bastion of psychoanalytic teaching and practice. So, in general, it had always been psychoanalysts, not just regular psychiatrists, who held power, influence, and territory (such as hospital beds, office and clinic space, and hours of the residents' time). How would these perquisites fare under Sachar, an enfant terrible of American psychiatry, who was just forty-three years old when he arrived to chair the institute. Though trained as an analyst, Sachar was famous for his research linking the brain and the endocrine system. For example, he was among the first to describe elevated levels of cortisol in the bloodstream of people with depression. This finding was at the time revolutionary, as it revealed a basic biological abnormality in people with an important psychiatric condition. To make matters worse, as far as the analysts were concerned, Sachar was bringing with him a band of fellow crusaders to help implement his mission—to make psychiatry evidence-based and biological, in line with other branches of medicine. It amounted to a biological invasion.

Paradoxically, this sea change suited me. I had no foreknowledge of these political shifts; nor did I know much about the history of the institute—simply that it was a large, prestigious place, as evidenced by the handsome brochure sent to all residency applicants. My ignorance may seem odd, but as I did not have the luxury of being able to visit the United States to scope out the different residencies ahead of time, Leora and I had to make big decisions based on small bits of data—like the glossiness of the brochure.

In South Africa at the time, psychiatry was considered necessary only for people with diseased minds. For the rest, according to this philosophy, people should sort out their own embarrassing problems, with the help of their families if necessary, but certainly out of the public eye. As for those who didn't have diseased minds but still sought out psychiatrists—well, they were probably just a bunch of self-absorbed Moaning Minnies with too much time and money on their hands. It was an unfortunate perspective, and one (I am sorry to say) that I also held to no small degree. So I welcomed Sachar and his band. Others feared the invaders, notably one of Sachar's chief aides, Donald Klein, another leading figure in U.S. psychiatry. In introducing Klein to the department, Sachar said, "Now, he's not going to be the Big Bad Wolf, but he's not going to be Good Time Charlie either." I doubt whether these words were any consolation to those who thought the former description far more accurate.

I was insufficiently sensitive to the fact that many others did not share my enthusiasm for the new regime, as became apparent when I met the supervisor who would oversee my work with long-term psychotherapy patients. At our first meeting, my supervisor asked me what my interests were. I replied honestly but naively that I wanted to do research on the biological bases of psychiatric illnesses. He was visibly furious that he had been assigned a lemon. His face turned white and his hands trembled as he took off his glasses and put them in their case.

"Then why on earth did you come to Columbia?" he asked, explaining to me its august psychoanalytic tradition.

Had I fully understood the dynamics at work in the institute, I would have answered more tactfully. As it was, I seemed to make matters worse with each response.

After we went to and fro a few times, I said to him, "Excuse me, but you seem very angry at this whole matter."

"Not that I'm aware of!" he shot back crisply.

So much for insight, I thought to myself (finally shutting up).

In retrospect I feel bad for putting the man in a difficult spot, but apparently he forgot about it, because some years later, at a Columbia reunion, he greeted me with the smile of an old friend, and said how proud he was whenever he saw me or my work featured in journals or the media.

Besides my regular residency work, I undertook a research project in the Lithium Clinic, which fell under the aegis of Ron Fieve, a pioneer in the use of lithium for bipolar disorder in the United States.

Now, Fieve had a beautiful suite of offices on the eleventh floor of the original institute building, which offered a commanding view of the vast Hudson River, with its slow-flowing waters and the majestic New Jersey Palisades across the way. It was clear from the start that Sachar could think of many things to do with those offices other than have

Fieve enjoy them. I got the scuttlebutt from Fieve's secretary, who, like all good secretaries, identified completely with her boss and his cause. "We're fighters here," she said. "We're not just going to roll over and play dead." Fieve himself confirmed this position to me. "He's taking on more than he knows," he told me on one occasion. "Like Eloise at the Plaza, I have resources. And do you know who the ultimate winner will be?" he asked. I didn't know whether it was a rhetorical question or not, so I waited. "The winner will be the last man left standing."

In academic institutions, if you want to get rid of someone and can't fire that person for some technical reason (like that dreadful nuisance called tenure), you take away that person's resources, go after his people, and make him as miserable as possible. As best I could tell, that was what Sachar was trying to do to Fieve, some of whose people were soon dispatched to a disused cavelike space in the bowels of the building. It would have made a good nesting place for bats or swiftlets.

On one occasion, I went to visit a friend from Fieve's group in his new digs with a glum expression on his face. "Look at me," he said, "here in my bunker, like Hitler."

"Without even the comforts of an Eva Braun," I countered, eliciting a wan smile.

Meanwhile, Sid Malitz, the formerly powerful acting director who had welcomed us residents like the paterfamilias, now became a ghost-like figure. His private patients would sit on a special chair at the end of a hallway, close to his new (much smaller) office. I remembered his kindness on that first day of residency and greeted him warmly whenever I saw him. Some sort of deal appeared to have been struck, by which he was allowed to keep an office and see his patients in exchange for remaining inconspicuous.

The analysts as a group were under siege. The most powerful of these, at least from the residents' point of view, was Roger MacKinnon, an outstanding teacher. I recall many of his lessons to this day. For example, of the unconscious mind, he had this to say: "You cannot see it directly. It's like the wind. You can only infer what it is doing by observing its effects on the branches of the trees." Previously feared and re-vered, MacKinnon had now fallen from institutional grace. Whereas formerly his lectures had been packed, now they were poorly attended. On one occasion, when I was the only resident there, he asked, "Where is everyone?"

I chose to answer the question concretely: "Jacobs is in the clinic, Coleman is at the community center," et cetera, et cetera.

"Of course I know that everyone can be accounted for," he said im-patiently. "The question is, why aren't they *here*?"

This time I chose not to answer. We both knew why they weren't there: MacKinnon had lost power, so people no longer thought it im-portant to attend his lectures. Surprisingly, I had begun to develop increasing respect for the analysts. Their theories might not explain bipolar disorder, but they certainly had a body of wisdom about dealing with patients. They understood the importance of the connection be-tween therapist and patient, and they knew how to foster and use that connection therapeutically. They had many valuable insights, which I wanted to learn to use. To my surprise, under their expert supervision, my own psychotherapy patients actually started to get better. Slowly, I began to shed my South African prejudices about therapy, which I would later seek out myself to good effect.

Overall, it seemed to me that the biologists and analysts both had much to offer. Was the clash of the titans really necessary? I wondered. Perhaps because of my lowly status as a resident, I was able to befriend people from both camps, benefit from their strengths and wisdom, and enjoy their mentorship.

In the end, I was invited to stay on at Columbia, but I was deter-mined that my future lay at the National Institute of Mental Health, which was then famous for its research training program. So I bade them all farewell. When I stopped off to see Ed Sachar, who was normally interpersonally awkward and unavailable, he was surprisingly warm. "Where do you think the future of psychiatry lies?" I asked him, knowing the question to be rather broad. "I don't know where it lies," he said. "But wherever it is, I'm sure you'll be there." It was like a father's blessing, and it meant a lot to me.

For years after moving to Bethesda, Maryland, I stayed in touch with my friends at the Psychiatric Institute. Tragedy hit Ed Sachar in the form of a stroke that left him paralyzed and aphasic. It was heartbreaking to see this brilliant and articulate man sitting in a wheelchair, struggling to communicate. Sid Malitz was once again drafted into service as acting director and given a research program of his own to run. Roger MacKinnon reemerged as a popular and respected teacher. As for Ron Fieve, he was, as he predicted, "the last man standing," and stayed on at the institute for years. Ed Sachar died tragically in 1984 at the age of fifty-one, only eight years after his meteoric ascent to the chair of psychiatry at the institute. Over the years, I have mentioned his name to several young psychiatrists; they have never heard of him. It is sobering to think that man so renowned in his time could fall into obscurity—like Ozymandias—just three decades after his triumphant conquest at Columbia.

> *Fortune is fickle. Be generous in victory and dignified in defeat.*

Chapter 27

Supervising a Supervisor

Be kind whenever possible.
It is always possible.
—THE DALAI LAMA

In my first year of residency, I was assigned a severe but brilliant supervisor, whose method of teaching was to rip my written presentations to shreds, finding nothing but defects. He must have sensed my discomfort, because he asked me at the beginning of one of our supervisory sessions whether something was off. I told him I had a migraine. "Does it have something to do with the supervision?" he asked—an excellent question, which I was not about to let pass. I told him that, indeed, nobody had ever found my writing so lacking in every respect, and that I found it very discouraging that he had nothing but criticism for my work.

Something seemed to register. He apologized, saying that learning ought to be fun, not torture. Henceforth he would take a different approach.

Well, I have never seen such a transformation. From that day on he became warm, kind, and extraordinarily helpful. I learned an enormous amount from him and he became one of my favorite teachers of all time. I developed a great trust in him and even consulted him on personal matters, about which he was invariably helpful.

After I left Columbia, our friendship continued to grow. We attend each other's major birthdays and make sure to stay in touch. At the time of writing, we have been friends for thirty-six years. I once asked him what had caused the turnaround in his behavior toward me during the residency. "Nobody had ever spoken to me the way you did," he said. "It made me reflect on myself and my teaching style, and I decided there must be a better way."

Some years later, I myself was managing a research group at the National Institute of Mental Health when a budget crisis occurred. A reduction in force was mandated, and according to some arcane government ruling, certain laid-off workers were allowed to "bump" other workers out of their positions. Through such a personnel shuffle, I ended up with Mark, a former manager, working under me as a research assistant.

Mark was a highly competent person, and as the days passed, I gave him task after task, as I was accustomed to do, and he tried his best to turn the work around. After a few weeks, however, he came to me and told me that he could not keep up with the number of tasks I was giving him. Would I be kind enough, he asked, to prioritize the work? Then he could make sure he accomplished the most important tasks by the end of the day or week.

I found this feedback useful. Previously, I had never thought about whether the work I was assigning could actually be done in the time allotted. Since nobody had asked this question before, I now began to wonder how my other research assistants had set their priorities, absent sufficient clarity from me. Some might have prioritized tasks according to their preferences, not the importance of the work. Others probably left work undone, either hoping I would not notice or simply picking it up when I did. And perhaps there were a few who took care to *look* busy, but were in fact bored and idle. I began to ask myself, How much *was* it reasonable to assign to a single assistant? And I made sure to spread the work out more evenly across the staff. In short, Mark's feedback made me a better manager with a happier staff. Once again, the supervisor had been supervised, except that this time I was the supervisor.

A final example of this general principle comes from one of my patients, Jim, a self-possessed high school senior who played lacrosse. According to Jim, his lacrosse coach had a harsh and punitive manner, which Jim found off-putting. The man was so rough it actually made him play worse. So, after trying to excel despite the coach, Jim ventured to offer some feedback: He told the coach that his critical style was affecting his game for the worse, but that he would be very responsive to a more encouraging and constructive approach. To the coach's credit, he was able to take in what Jim said and use it to turn around the relationship. As you might expect, not only did Jim's game improve but also that of the whole team.

All three stories have several things in common: a subordinate who is willing to speak up and does so respectfully, an open-minded supervisor, and a happy ending. If the subordinate is rude or the supervisor pigheaded, a happy ending is unlikely. On the other hand, if conditions are favorable, this approach is worth a try.

> *Don't let your position in a hierarchy define you. Analyze your situation and make a thoughtful judgment about your supervisor. If you proceed with courtesy and respect, you may be able to influence a system favorably from the bottom up.*

Chapter 28

What Are the Questions? Becoming a Researcher

"What is the answer?" asked Gertrude Stein shortly
before her death, as she was being wheeled into the
operating room.

Alice B. Toklas was silent.

"In that case," Stein asked, "what is the question?"

As a budding researcher, newly attached to Frederick Goodwin's research group at the National Institute of Mental Health (NIMH),
I was finally in a position to start fulfilling my longtime dream: to
discover something that would make a difference to people with emotional problems. But what should I tackle? It struck me that throughout
my schooling, I had been presented with questions, which I was expected to answer correctly. Now I had to find my own questions, to
which the answers should be significant—and provable—but not yet
known. It seemed like a tall order. There were many researchers on
Goodwin's unit, but I gravitated toward those specializing in circadian

rhythms, the body's own internal clocks, which appeared to be abnormal in many people with mood disorders.

The way it worked, senior researchers would approach us new recruits with ideas they thought we might like to work on or, more commonly, that they would like to have us work on. So it was that I was directed to a potential new antidepressant. The drug ultimately became Wellbutrin (bupropion), a highly successful antidepressant, but I do not regret declining the project. I reasoned that even if the drug worked, there wouldn't be much excitement in moving yet another compound from the lab to the patient. Another drug suggested to me as a potentially novel antidepressant was a powerful new opiate. Once again, this idea failed to excite. I reasoned that opiates had been around for centuries, and none had been effective and dependable as antidepressants. Why should this one be different?

So it was that I declined one potential study after another. Putting activity monitors on people with manic depression? Too predictable. They would of course be more active during mania and less so during depression. Systematically telling night owls to go to bed on time? If that would help, patients (or their mothers) would have long since figured it out. No, I wanted to "take a flier," an expression that had been passed down through the NIMH over generations of researchers, as chronicled in Robert Kanigel's *Apprentice to Genius.*

Some of the patients residing on the clinical unit where I worked suffered from rapid-cycling bipolar disorder. These people alternated between manic and depressed states with alarming frequency. Typically, they remained in one state for no longer than about two weeks, sometimes much less. I wondered whether there might be some chemical that was oversecreted during mania and undersecreted during depression. What would happen, I wondered, if I drew a pint of blood from someone in a manic state, spun off the red cells, froze the plasma, and transfused it back to the same person in a depressed state? It speaks well for the NIMH that such a far-out study was supported. I ran a few people through the protocol but observed zero benefit. In retrospect, that is no surprise, as I was making far too many assumptions: First, that such a substance existed; second, that it would enter the blood in detectable concentrations; third, that it would survive freezing and thawing; fourth, that it would reenter the brain in sufficient amounts after transfusion; and so on. It was a flier that flopped.

Then I wondered whether perhaps the greatest discoveries in neuroscience would emerge from the laboratory. Could it be that in working with patients, I was hunting for clues in the wrong place? A very talented senior colleague kindly offered to mentor me in his lab, where I set about analyzing blood elements called platelets, taken from people with depression versus healthy controls. I also conducted studies with rats. I soon became bored with platelets and allergic to rats. My mentor helped soften the pain of my leaving by observing that I was "a bit klutzy" for that sort of work anyway.

All these setbacks, however, turned out to be good news. They helped me recognize that I had chosen psychiatry because it dealt with *people*. From my earliest years, I had spent time studying people in order to understand their thoughts and feelings. I enjoyed working with *people*—not platelets and rats. So it made sense that my research should center on my clinical work, regardless of where the most glittering prizes were to be found.

I have heard that entrepreneurs trying to found start-up companies are advised to fail frequently. The rationale is that trying many different things is the best way to find out which holds the most promise. Likewise, young CEOs are told not to linger too long on anything that isn't working. In retrospect, I followed these general principles from the start of my research career: I tried many things in order to see where best to put my efforts.

Years later, when I was traveling in a plane over the Alps, I asked the friend and fellow researcher sitting next to me, "Alex, what is the next best question to ask?" He answered wryly, "Sometimes it's a challenge simply not to ask the wrong question." Many a researcher will identify with that statement. We have all wasted time asking questions that turn out, after a long and arduous slog, to lead nowhere or to generate only trivial results.

Shortly before my arrival at the NIMH, in the late 1970s, my colleagues Alfred Lewy and Thomas Wehr had shown that the normal nighttime secretion of melatonin into the bloodstream could be suppressed by exposing people to bright artificial light. This discovery turned out to be extremely important, because until that time, when it came to humans, scientists had considered environmental light simply in terms of its visual effects. People needed light in order to see: end of story. This new finding indicated, for the first time in humans, that light might have nonvisual effects as well. Melatonin is a hormone secreted by the pineal gland, a pea-size structure tucked under the brain, which some modern scientists had thought was a vestigial remnant without a function. Now we were wondering whether the pineal gland might actually help regulate sleep and circadian rhythms.

In order to explain how Lewy and Wehr's discovery led me to my future explorations, I should tell you two more things about melatonin. First, scientists have long known that melatonin helps mediate the effects of the seasons, at least in animals: It influences a whole range of behaviors in species from single-celled algae all the way to sheep and cattle. It now seems as though we may be able to add humans to that list. For a discussion of these effects, I refer the interested reader to my book *Winter Blues.* Second, the neural pathways that trigger the suppression of melatonin by light are well understood. After light reaches the eye, stimuli travel from the retina through the hypothalamus, a primitive—and therefore fundamental—part of the brain. Then, after a roundabout passage through the neck, they go all the way back up to the pineal gland. The hypothalamus regulates basic functions such as appetite, weight, and daily rhythms, all of which may be disturbed in people with depression.

So here was a neural pathway that might explain how the changing seasons affect mood: by the seasonal waxing and waning of sunlight. It was a radical notion at the time. Pioneering scientist Louis Pasteur said that chance favors the prepared mind—and my mind was certainly prepared, because by then Leora and I had suffered through three or four winter depressions while living in the United States, all of which had resolved in the summer. Those months of misery were soon to yield dividends.

Another crucial stimulus was the arrival at the NIMH of a sixty-three-year-old scientist named Herb Kern, who had noticed seasonal cycles of depression going back many years. Since he was a physicist and not a psychiatrist, Herb was unencumbered by psychological theories. Instead, he simply looked at his own data—piles of small journals he had kept for years—saw that his dark moods came and went with the shorter and longer days, and hypothesized that seasonal changes in day length could be the trigger.

That winter, Wehr, Lewy, and I treated Herb by exposing him to bright light for two hours in the morning and again in the evening—times when he would ordinarily have been exposed only to regular room light. As predicted, he snapped out of his depression and stayed well for months.

Was Herb a curiosity? Was this a rare form of mood disorder or were there others like him? My own experience suggested the latter, and one colleague in private practice said he had observed others with seasonal mood problems. In order to investigate a treatment, however, you have to conduct a controlled experiment, for which you need a group of patients. A wise old mentor once told me a rule that applies to all clinical research: No patients, no study. So . . . where might I find enough patients? When I polled local psychiatrists, they all denied ever having seen people who became depressed every winter.

Nowadays, with people all over the world routinely using bright lights all winter long, those colleagues might seem, in retrospect, a bit dim. I should remind you in their defense, however, that the idea of darkness and light affecting moods was at the time a new paradigm. It was natural, given their training, that my colleagues should see their patients' depressions as triggered by events in their lives—a distant spouse, a setback at work, an ailing parent—all no doubt important, but not necessarily the *cause* of their depression. Some might even be the *effects* of their depression. To complicate matters further, the depressed person casts about for explanations—and finds them. As one of my patients put it, a depressed person will always find some reason to be depressed. You can imagine how, with all these "causes" in play, the biggest culprit—the lack of sunlight—could easily be missed. In a way, the effect was so big it was hard to see.

Since doctors did not recognize seasonal depression, my only recourse was to appeal to the people themselves. So I did something now routine but then thought tacky (right up there with an ambulance-chasing lawyer): I advertised for patients, because otherwise there would be no patients and no study. Luckily, a *Washington Post* reporter was intrigued enough to write an article about a young woman who had suffered regular winter depressions. "I should have been a bear," the woman said, "because bears are allowed to hibernate. Humans are not." The article drew thousands of responses from all over the country, including many from the local area. The mail lay in heaps all over my desk, and I have seldom been so happy.

We recruited our patients in the summer, when they were well, and, as luck would have it, although other researchers were also trying to conduct studies in the clinical rooms at that time, they did not have many patients. So Wehr and I had all the rooms we needed. The place was full of our patients, all looking disconcertingly happy and carefree—not what you expect on a psychiatric unit. Skeptical colleagues asked me, "What if they don't become depressed? Won't you look stupid?" But I had a powerful hunch that they *would* become depressed. And besides, years of fumbling around with a cricket bat had taught me that looking stupid is not the worst thing in the world.

Autumn arrived, the days grew shorter, the leaves took on their splendid glowing colors, and, one by one, just as they had predicted, our patients began to develop their fall-winter symptoms. It was a supremely exciting moment. I felt as though I were witnessing a law of nature, an ingrained response to the seasons that had been around for all of human time, yet never seen before through this lens. It recalled to mind the famous lines by John Keats:

> *Then felt I like some watcher of the skies*
> *When a new planet swims into his ken;*
> *Or like stout Cortez when with eagle eyes*
> *He star'd at the Pacific—and all his men*
> *Look'd at each other with a wild surmise—*
> *Silent, upon a peak in Darien.*

I had found my question, and dozens of questions followed—naturally and easily, as happens when science is flowing in the right direction.

The results were not universally accepted, of course. They may well have seemed too good to be true, or too strange. Even after Wehr and I had published a description of the condition, which we called seasonal affective disorder (SAD), and had shown in a controlled study that bright light could reverse its symptoms, some colleagues laughed. It took perseverance to establish the new form of depression and the new treatment alongside the others in the canon. What gave me the conviction to hang in there, besides my observations and the replication studies that began to appear, were my own personal experiences that light and dark definitely had power to transform my own mood.

> *If you wish to find the best answers, ask the right questions.*
> *Then find the right employer and colleagues.*

Chapter 29

Leaving the NIMH

When the curtain falls, it is time to get off the stage.

—JOHN MAJOR, BRITISH PRIME MINISTER, 1990–1997

No one can make you feel inferior without your consent.

—ELEANOR ROOSEVELT, U.S. FIRST LADY, 1933–1945

spent more than twenty years at the NIMH—good years, for the most
part. The seasons came and went quickly, and always, it seemed, there
were new questions to ask, new studies to do. We defined the syndrome
of seasonal affective disorder and described its typical symptom profile:
depression, plus other features, such as overeating, oversleeping, craving sweets and starches, and weight gain. We estimated its frequency at
different latitudes and found, as you might expect, that it is more and
more common as you go farther north. Importantly, we also documented and treated SAD in children and adolescents, among whom it
is quite common and especially easy to miss, because parents and teachers *expect* teenagers to be moody. Untreated, SAD takes a serious toll on
their enjoyment of their school days and college life, not to mention

their studies and their expectations of what a "normal" life should be like.

Tom Wehr and I also encountered people who described an opposite pattern of SAD, in which they became depressed in summer and felt better in winter. As you might guess, this pattern of summer SAD is more common as you get closer to the equator. Although depressed and unproductive like their winter counterparts, people with summer SAD often tend to sleep and eat *less* and to *lose* weight during summer— just the opposite of those with winter SAD. Also, people with summer SAD are more likely to be agitated (rather than slowed down), and to have more suicidal thoughts than those with classic SAD. Although Wehr and I speculated as to what environmental factors might trigger these summer depressions, we did not find a satisfactory answer. We hypothesized that too much of either heat or light might trigger and maintain their symptoms, but were unable to find a "cold therapy" or "dark therapy" that was as effective as light for winter SAD.

Wehr put activity monitors on people with rapid-cycling bipolar disorder to assess their activity level as they switched between manic and depressed states. The tracings revealed that a sleepless night often occurred just before a person switched from depression into mania. Aside from our research, Wehr and I also had private practices, which often fed our research with good ideas. Each of us had in our practice a patient who regularly became manic the very day after a sleepless night, as did another colleague in our group, David Sack. My patient was typical: a college student in Florida, who would drive home to Maryland straight through the night. On arriving home, he invariably became manic. Wehr, Sack, and I combined our experiences with our three patients and wrote a paper called "Sleep Deprivation as a Final Common Pathway in the Genesis of Mania." This paper influenced the standard treatment of bipolar disorder, so that proper sleep and maintaining regular circadian rhythms are now routinely emphasized.

Much of my research at the NIMH revolved around light therapy. We figured out, for example, that light therapy for SAD works via the eyes, not the skin; and many other details that are important for those who need this form of treatment. We found that light therapy can help people with conditions other than SAD—for example, premenstrual syndrome and abnormal circadian rhythms. The last group includes extreme late night owls, people who are unable to get to work on time. And finally, we conducted studies to determine what underlying anomalies in brain chemistry might explain why some people have seasonal depressions, while others don't. (Again, the details of all this research can be found in my book *Winter Blues*.)

My chief collaborator and best friend in all these projects was Tom Wehr, who was in fact my boss at the NIMH—though, for some strange reason, he never acted like a boss; nor did he feel like one. We met once a week to discuss ongoing research and anything else that happened to come up. Tom is widely read in many fields, though his passion was his research. While at the NIMH, he said he felt as if he were working in the garden of the Medicis, referring to the powerful family who patronized artists and scientists in Renaissance Florence. The person most responsible for supporting *our* work was Director Fred Goodwin, who believed in the value of what Tom and I were doing. We flourished both because of his support and, I like to believe, because the work itself was inherently valuable.

Value, however, is very much in the eye of the beholder. At the NIMH, as in any other institution, we saw people's fortunes rise and fall. There was a general sense, when someone's unit was shut down, that it was probably deserved, that the work must not have been good enough. The survivors took comfort in thinking that they were safe because their work was superior. I use the third person here, but no doubt I was guilty of the same self-serving thought patterns at times, even though I'd seen that all-out hostile takeover at Columbia, where many highly accomplished people were sidelined or forced out.

Now, at the NIMH, I saw a similar process. Those who had fallen from grace would wander the halls, looking downcast. Others generally avoided them, as though their misfortune might be contagious. I found this behavior both intriguing and disgusting. I remembered my friends and those I had admired at Columbia when they fell from grace. That fall did not change who they were as people or what they had to offer. I made it my business to befriend those who suffered institutional reversals. I have no idea whether anyone noticed or appreciated my gestures, but they were my private protest against this type of shunning. I also realized (in a theoretical sort of way) that one day the person in disfavor might just as easily be me.

Researchers at the NIMH were judged periodically (in our day, every four years) by a group of outside investigators called the Board of Scientific Counselors (BSC). Judgment by one's peers is, of course, both reasonable and necessary. What I didn't know (and nobody tells you) is that the judgment is heavily loaded to ensure the outcome desired by the institute director. That worked well for our group when the director supported our work. One early BSC was loaded with people I had known from Columbia and others favorably disposed to our work. The evening before the review, the NIMH put on a festive dinner for both counselors and counseled. One of the counselors, a friend of mine who was seated at my table, said, "Isn't there something odd about this? You're giving aid and comfort to the enemy." After dinner, when Fred Goodwin addressed the visitors, he praised our group in a way that left no doubt that he wanted to continue to support us. One counselor (I'll call him Dr. M) shouted out from the back of the room, "It's okay, Fred. I know my job," meaning that he had already been briefed to turn in a positive review, so enough with the praise already. The review went well and I was granted tenure.

Years passed, Fred left his leadership role, and in due course we acquired a new director (I'll call him Dr. A, as in ax). In retrospect, especially to a veteran of the hostile takeover at Columbia, it should have been obvious that his mission was to "cut out the deadwood" and "turn the institution around." Too bad we didn't know it at the time. Tom and I were surprised, but not worried, that Dr. A showed no interest in our work. We assumed that his attention was needed elsewhere. His priority soon emerged, however: It was to jettison a bunch of senior researchers and sequester their budgets and positions; then he'd have the resources to attract a Big Fish, who could be promised enough positions to staff an entire research department.

We didn't clearly see it coming, though, for a few reasons: First, we believed that science would dictate policy, and that we had proved our worth; second, we foolishly believed that the BSC process was fair; but most important, we had been too comfortable for too long. We had been basking like the giant tortoises of the Galápagos, who had no natural predators—until humans arrived on the scene.

On the morning of our next BSC review, I woke up with a migraine. I had never before woken up with a migraine, so I took it as a bad omen (which it was). Needless to say, there had been no festive dinner the night before. Leora rushed out to the emergency pharmacy to get me medicine, which silenced the little men playing congas in my cranium. When I got to the room where the review was to occur, they were waiting for me. A chief attack dog had been appointed, and he carried out his mission faithfully. His demeanor was vicious—unlike any to which I had previously been subjected in a review. It was obvious that he had no genuine interest in the work, only its deficiencies. It was the behavior of someone who wanted to ax, not to inquire or promote discussion. At the back of the hall sat Dr. A, chatting and snickering with his cronies, clearly uninterested in the proceedings and feeling no need to pretend otherwise.

Shortly afterward, not surprisingly, word came down that my group would be dismantled. I would be able to work on till I was eligible for retirement, which was the least they could do, given that I had tenure so could not legally be fired (except for cause).

I had mixed reactions. I was deeply angry at the injustice of the review itself. It had never been my sense that judgments about research at a premier U.S. institution could be so biased—imperfect, of course, as human judgments always are, but not a priori partisan. I was wrong.

At the same time, apart from my anger, another sense began to stir within me. As the weeks passed, I became aware that I had actually ceased to feel excited at the NIMH. So maybe moving on would be okay. Maybe, just maybe, it was a good time to go.

Over the years, several colleagues had tried to recruit me to their psychiatric departments, but I had always declined. The work was flowing, and I felt productive. Now I remembered that one of these colleagues had said to me, "In order to leave, you need both a push and a pull. Right now, you have no push." Well, now I'd had a push. Perhaps the BSC, without intending to, had done me a favor.

It was one thing to want to leave, however, and another to be booted out so unjustly and unceremoniously. I had two personal friends on the BSC, who confirmed my perception that the group had been gunning for me from the start. I smile now as I think of my naïveté, but I was truly shocked that a group of scientists would so willingly yield to an administrator's bidding.

It reminds me of my naïveté many years before, when I assumed that all schoolteachers were perfect spellers. Now I realize, more in sorrow than in anger, that scientists are like everyone else. While most are honest and principled, some are partisan and corruptible.

I stopped myself from brooding by recalling Sid Malitz, the acting director at Columbia, and other colleagues who had maintained their dignity in the face of reversals of fortune, and I drew strength from their examples. Likewise, I remembered my colleague Norio Ozaki, a brilliant Japanese psychiatrist who had worked as a fellow in our unit when suddenly, for no good reason, his visa was withdrawn. We appealed the decision, but were powerless to reverse it. Angry on his behalf, I explained the situation to Norio, who responded simply and with great serenity, "Sometimes life is like that." Norio is now the chair of psychiatry at Nagoya University in Japan.

I concluded that unfairness is just one more type of adversity—something to learn from. I would seek to emulate Malitz's dignity and Norio's serenity. Furthermore, I would use the downturn as a stimulus to creativity and pursue another childhood dream of mine—to write.

I was by no means alone in being axed. The director's goal, after all, was to accumulate a pool of positions for the Big Fish. So yet more people had to be culled. As the process unfolded, one senior scientist observed, "We used to be smart; now we're dumb."

Some found ways to fight back. Eminent neuroscientist Paul Mac-Lean, who was very senior when he appeared before the BSC in the last years of his career, actually poked fun at the reviewers. He opened with a complaint that they should not hold meetings in the daytime during boating season. Then he went on to advance a theory that Homo sapiens had crossbred with Neanderthals somewhere along the line (which now appears to be true). Evidence, MacLean said, could be found in the form of bumps on the skull in the progeny of such cross-breeding. He then went about palpating the skulls of the counselors until he claimed to find someone with the right type of bump, and exclaimed with glee, "Ah, here we have one!" It probably made no difference to the outcome, but it must have felt good.

Another colleague fought back (with teeth) when he learned that one of the counselors who panned his work actually had a financial conflict of interest in the work under review, which he had not disclosed. Such an egregious omission flunks what D.C. insiders call "the *Washington Post* smell test," and the scientist thereby earned lasting immunity from subsequent BSC attack. Unfortunately, it is not always possible to demonstrate bias, even when it is there. Incidentally, the corrupt counselor in question had previously approached Tom and promised a favorable review if Tom would request him as a counselor. Tom, of course, had declined.

To top it off, remember the Big Fish (I'll call him Dr. B), the one who would eventually acquire the cache of positions? Well, he was right there during my BSC review, sitting next to the director and conferring with him. A conflict of interest? Not at all, Dr. B reassured Tom sometime after the review—though he conceded that it might be viewed as such.

Well, after a few weeks of fuming, I was through with the matter—or so I thought. I secured a contract to write a book on the herbal antidepressant St. John's wort, for which I obtained all the permissions necessary for "outside activities." When word got out, though, I got a letter from the acting scientific director, telling me in a cheerful tone that I had taken on a very "controversial" topic. She was sure I didn't want any unpleasantness, she wrote, so everybody's interests would be served if I ceased and desisted: no more St. John's wort. That was the last straw! I did not emigrate from apartheid South Africa to the United States in order to be told what I could or could not write. I wrote back that I had no intention of following her instructions. I had the written permissions, and the kangaroo court to which I had been subjected had made it clear they simply wanted me gone. If so, I suggested that *they* cease and desist: no more harassment. Then I could get on with my transition to my new life. I showed Tom the letter, to which he said, "Good. Sometimes it's better to be part of the problem than part of the solution."

The next day the lawyer for the institute called me, full of blandishments and placatory comments. Apparently they got my message: If they wanted me to go quietly, they should leave me alone.

Tom and I were both moved to proverbial "broom closet" offices. When Leora stopped by, she laughed and said, "How humiliating." I laughed back, not feeling humiliated because I was too busy moving on.

To any seasoned NIH administrator, it was clear that Tom would be next to go. "That's how they manage you out," a knowledgeable friend told me. "First they get rid of the people under you, thereby destroying your ability to produce anything. Then they ax you for not being productive—or for some other reason." And that's exactly what happened to Tom at his next review. And so the institute lost, for no good reason, one of the most creative, accomplished, and knowledgeable clinical researchers who had ever graced its halls, while he was still in the prime of his career.

WHEN I INTERVIEWED TOM for this piece, he said, very kindly, "Your genuine interest in the research, in being inclusive and developing the field, did not prepare you for the cynical game of power that many play. In order to succeed at that game, you have to shift gears and think of your career as a power game, which some people do all the time. But you didn't want to shift gears. So there was no way to win at that game."

It must have been for the best, I told Tom, because there has not been a day since leaving the NIMH that I have woken up and wished I were back there. He agreed, adding, "The place I had worked in ceased to exist, and that made it easier to leave. I didn't like the place it had become."

I HAVE WRITTEN about the final chapter of my story at the NIMH because this kind of thing happens to many people in all fields, and is relevant to the subject of the book—adversity and how best to deal with it. Sometimes life is like that. Sometimes you need to accept that it's time to move on—and to do so.

Notwithstanding the bumpy ending, my overwhelming feeling about my time at the NIMH is gratitude—for the collaborations with gifted colleagues and inspiring patients, for the thrill to see with fresh eyes the laws of nature unfolding, and to discover new influences of light and dark on human behavior. It was a supreme privilege to work and play in such good company and for so many years in the garden of the Medicis.

> *Look within to gauge your worth rather than depending on institutions or the opinions of others, for institutions rise and fall, and fashions come and go, but a good sense of your own value will see you through life's ups and downs.*

Chapter 30

Losing and Choosing

The art of losing isn't hard to master.

—ELIZABETH BISHOP

Two roads diverged in a wood, and I—
I took the one less traveled by,
And that has made all the difference.

—ROBERT FROST

When I arrived at Columbia, shortly after leaving South Africa, I decided to undertake a project for our residency group—to assemble a set of poems that dealt with the death of a parent. One of my supervisors, who had lost both parents as a young girl, thought the choice a strange one. It does not seem so to me, however. I had just left my home country, where I knew I would never live again. My father was seriously ill, and I knew I might never see him again either. Although excited to be in New York City and studying pure psychiatry at last, I was grappling with feelings of loss. To deal with these feelings, I turned to what has been a dependable comfort for me—poetry.

In putting my project together, I was assisted by a memorable accomplice—a brilliant secretary, who took a particular interest, as she herself had been orphaned at a young age. In attempting to empathize, I told her that I too dreaded the prospect of losing my parents. "You will never experience," she said, "the kind of pain a child experiences on losing a parent. It is very different when you are an adult." She was right, of course. Research shows that such an early loss can be devastating, making it difficult for children to develop emotional attachments to others; the children are also more susceptible to depression in later life.

Loss is, of course, a huge subject, and great tomes have been devoted to its many aspects. In this short piece, I would like to focus on one particular aspect of loss: realizing that the loss has occurred, which is an essential first step. Only after we *get* it can we come to terms with it.

One sunny day in Midtown Manhattan, Leora, Josh, and I were out walking with friends when we spotted a man selling helium-filled Mylar balloons. Such balloons are commonplace now, but then they were a high-end item, so we all viewed it as a great extravagance when one of our friends insisted on buying one for Josh. It was spectacular—large, glittering, and silver as it bobbed along, reflecting the fancy store windows that lined the streets.

Josh held on to the balloon for a few blocks, then declared that he wanted to let it go. I protested, saying that was no way to treat a gift, and did he understand that once he let go, the balloon would drift away and he could never get it back? Yes, Josh said, he understood. He just wanted to see what would happen if he let it go. "Let him do it," said the extravagant friend. "Why not?" And so he did.

At that moment, my feelings about Josh's decision shifted. No longer the thrifty parent, I joined in the celebration, along with the friend who had cheered Josh along. I will never forget the sight of that round silvery pod drifting up, up, up past the skyscrapers into the perfect blue Manhattan sky, the buildings reflected in its polished surfaces and the sun glinting off its crenellated seam. I understood how wise Josh had been, and our friend for encouraging him. As a consequence, we were left with an indelible image of perfection—far better than a half-deflated old balloon knocking about the apartment till someone finally threw it out.

The incident with the balloon has often served as an image that helps me let something go. Confronted with the prospect of losing someone or something I value dearly, I summon up the balloon and the feelings that went through my mind in relation to it—minor panic at the idea of loss, the moment of acceptance, the memory of its brief shimmering perfection. These recollections have stayed with me all these years, and whatever it is I am about to lose, they help me . . . let it go.

Another image I have used for letting go comes from an Impressionist painting I once saw, a Manet perhaps, in which a small boat is moored in a river, floating in the dappled shade of a willow. There are a few people in it—I can't remember the details. Perhaps they're having a picnic or spending an intimate hour. In any event, sometimes when I am having difficulty letting go of someone or something, I mentally put the lost whatever in the boat, untie the moorings, and watch the boat drift gently down the river and out of sight.

The key to both little dramas is that you are making a conscious choice. The first step is to acknowledge and feel the beauty and value of whatever is being lost. The second step is to deliberately let it go, using an image that works for you. This process is a way to reclaim a feeling of control in a situation where you may not have much (if any) control. I will tell you more about this way of thinking in the chapter on my meeting with the great Viktor Frankl, who said that in a situation in which you have no control—in his case Auschwitz—the one thing you *can* control is the attitude you choose to take. Imagery is one way to help you shift your view of things.

I have at times shared these techniques with patients, one of whom discovered a useful variant: You can also choose to lose something unpleasant. The woman in question was furious with her husband for having had an affair, and even more furious with the object of his desire. Although the affair was long past, she was having difficulty letting go of her rage. "Can you give me some imagery to help get rid of this woman from my mind?" she asked. I offered her the balloon and the boat, acknowledging that they seemed too paltry to assuage the intensity of her fury. Nevertheless, at the next session she told me that using imagery had been helpful. She had adapted the idea to a mountain slope, where she visualized her rival skiing into a dense fog until she disappeared—and plummeted off a cliff into oblivion. Although I don't recommend this particular variant, my patient was quite satisfied with the outcome of the exercise.

When confronted with serious loss, people often struggle to accept that the loss has in fact occurred. The writer Joan Didion communicates this poignantly in *The Year of Magical Thinking*, in which she documents the year following her husband's sudden death. She describes, for example, how she felt reluctant to get rid of his shoes; she kept thinking he might come back and need them, a type of magical thinking we see following all types of disasters.

After 9/11, for example, one father clung to the fact that his daughter, who worked in one of the towers, had called 911 at a specific time after the plane struck the building. She had been alive then! She had survived the crash! So the father thought that if only, if only he could trace her movements *after* the moment of the call, then perhaps his daughter would be found alive. His pleas for news of her were actually broadcast on TV, for even though it was obvious to everyone that the daughter was dead, nobody wanted to challenge his reasoning. There was a tacit understanding that this was a phase of mourning he had to slog through as best he could. This father could let go of hope only in his own time and his own way.

The basis for magical thinking, also known as denial, is an unconscious belief that if we don't face our loss, we won't have to take the hit and feel the pain. So we put it off. Obviously, denial can be sustained for only so long, because it is at odds with reality. This kind of thinking is caricatured in Road Runner cartoons, in which we see the same story again and again: the tall and scrawny bird is always chased by his enemy, Wile E. Coyote, who has some devious plot, such as to lure the bird onto a bomb. Yet the coyote always loses, often running full speed off the edge of a cliff—at which point common sense says the animal should immediately plunge into the abyss. Instead, he stays suspended, running in mid-air . . . until he looks down. Only then does he fall. In this visual joke, the coyote's denial keeps him safe, while accepting it leads to disaster. In the real world, it works the other way around.

Unfortunately, the inability to accept the loss of a relationship can take the extreme form of stalking, especially in those predisposed to controlling others or to violence. For example, I once knew a promising psychiatric resident who broke up with her boyfriend. From her point of view the relationship was over. From his, that outcome was impossible, inconceivable, unacceptable. So he took control in a pathological way: He stalked and killed her. It was a real-life version of the plot of the opera *Carmen*.

Loss of a significant person is painful, the loss of a loved one especially so. A friend once confided to me his deep unhappiness in the wake of such a loss. In trying to console him, I pointed out that losing is an art: You get better at it the more you practice, as you understand the stages through which grief takes you and learn how to deal with them. My friend, a fellow poetry enthusiast, became excited. "Do you know Elizabeth Bishop's poem 'One Art'?" he asked. I did not, but it has since become one of my all-time favorites. For those unfamiliar with this brilliant poem, here it is:

One Art

By Elizabeth Bishop

The art of losing isn't hard to master;
so many things seem filled with the intent
to be lost that their loss is no disaster.

Lose something every day. Accept the fluster
of lost door keys, the hour badly spent.
The art of losing isn't hard to master.

Then practice losing farther, losing faster:
places, and names, and where it was you meant
to travel. None of these will bring disaster.

I lost my mother's watch. And look! my last, or
next-to-last, of three loved houses went.
The art of losing isn't hard to master.

I lost two cities, lovely ones. And, vaster,
some realms I owned, two rivers, a continent.
I miss them, but it wasn't a disaster.

—Even losing you (the joking voice, a gesture
I love) I shan't have lied. It's evident
the art of losing's not too hard to master
though it may look like (Write it!) like disaster.

In advising us to practice losing, Bishop counsels acceptance of the loss itself—a fundamental first step to adjusting to it. She also reassures the reader that loss, however large (and she escalates the scale and impact as she goes), does not have to be a disaster. Most of us are programmed to survive, no matter how painful our loss may be. This survival capacity, evolved over millennia and embedded in our DNA, is buttressed by the support of family, friends, and community.

The formal structure that Bishop uses for her poem—the villanelle, with its rigid requirements for length and rhyme scheme—reminds me of the formal rituals that members of different religions use to help the mourners deal with death—such as an Irish wake or the Jewish practice of sitting shiva.

Most of us know, and social custom reinforces, the need to accept—in a real sense, to choose—the reality that someone has died or something is lost. Otherwise, we cannot heal. We are perhaps less aware of an important paired truth: that every major choice involves a loss.

How many of us have made a life choice, then wondered how it might have been had we gone another way: What if we'd married the other person? Studied another field? Settled in another place? I chose to leave South Africa and move to the United States, and in so doing, like so many millions of other immigrants, I left behind parents, family, and homeland. The choice to leave was, for us, a good one: I have always been sure of that. At the same time, the losses both large and small were real and had to be mourned. At some level I must have known that when I set about putting together the poems on loss for my residency class.

This universal experience of choice—of two roads, only one of which can be chosen—is brilliantly captured in Robert Frost's familiar poem "The Road Not Taken," which I quote at the head of the chapter.

The poem's proverbial fork in the road is an age-old, archetypal image for a choice. In the poem, Frost tells himself that he can always come back and explore the other path, but he understands that, "as way leads on to way," that is unlikely to happen. Any major choice is a commitment, at least to some extent, because even if you change your mind later, the new moment of choice and its circumstances will be different—and so will you. It is valuable, therefore, to appreciate that for every opportunity taken, an opportunity is lost.

Opportunity cost, a concept used in business, applies equally to other aspects of life. By making a choice, we forfeit alternative options. I should emphasize that I am not referring here to minor choices, which are easily reversed. In business, there is a maxim: "If a choice is easy to reverse, you can make it quickly. If it will be hard to reverse, take more time to think it over." The principle is useful in daily life as well.

At the end of the poem, Frost says that "ages hence," he will tell that he took the road less traveled by and that has made all the difference. I once heard the eminent scientist Stephen Jay Gould discuss this poem. He took issue with Frost's conclusion because initially, the poem says that the two paths had been worn to about the same degree. Gould thought that Frost was exaggerating the importance of the road less traveled—as perhaps many of us dramatize the importance of the choices we make and the lives we lead.

I see things otherwise: I agree with Frost. Whatever road a person takes is by definition the road less traveled, because we are each one of us on a unique journey. The paths we choose—and the gains and losses we sustain in taking those paths—shape the scope and contours of our lives. Our choices make us who we are.

> *The first step in coping with loss is to realize and accept that it has occurred. Then you can take the necessary measures to cope with it.*
>
> *Each significant choice we make involves both a commitment and a loss; so choose your path carefully at every major fork in the road, for the sum of your choices will shape your life.*

Chapter 31

Pride and Prejudice and Sociopaths

Prejudice is a great time saver. You can form opinions
without having to get the facts.

—E. B. WHITE

I have written about racial prejudice in apartheid South Africa, which
was rampant and extreme. As we know, however, the scourge of prejudice is not confined to far-off shores. The following story, told me by a
friend, is just one example.

A friend's uncle, Bill, a middle-aged white man living in Chicago,
was walking in the city late at night and had to cross a narrow bridge to
get home. He saw a black man approaching from the opposite direction
and realized he would have to brush up against this other man, and risk
having his wallet snatched. As the two men passed on the bridge, sure
enough, their arms brushed. Uncle Bill instantly put his hand into his
left pocket and, indeed, he found no wallet there. He turned on the
stranger angrily and shouted, "Give me that wallet." Then he reached

into the other man's pocket, felt a wallet, and grabbed it. The stranger fled. When Uncle Bill got home, he found he had two wallets—his own, which had been in his *right* pocket, and the other man's, which he had stolen.

The more I have traveled and the more people I know, the more I realize that prejudice is universal. Although the *degree* of prejudice in apartheid South Africa was extraordinary and institutionalized, the country also served as a convenient outlet for the wrath of people who might more usefully address the prejudice in their own schools, back-yards, and homes.

In this chapter, however, my focus is not on prejudice as a societal phenomenon but on aspects of its psychological roots; its appearance in Jane Austen's celebrated novel *Pride and Prejudice*; and its relevance to a particular group of people—psychopaths (also known as sociopaths).

In one of Aesop's fables, a lamb is drinking from the same river as a wolf. "Lamb," says the wolf, "you have contaminated my water. For that reason, I will have to eat you."

"But, Sir Wolf," replies the lamb, "it is impossible for me to have contaminated your water, for as you see, I am drinking downstream from you."

"Well, Lamb," says the wolf, "last year this time you *did* contaminate my drinking water. Therefore I will have to eat you."

"But, Sir Wolf," replies the lamb, "that is impossible. I am only six months old!"

"Well, in that case," said the wolf, "it must have been your father." And he gobbled up the lamb.

This fable has a modern counterpart in a tale that harks back to the "literacy tests" conducted in the certain parts of the United States right into the 1960s. These so-called tests were supposed to determine whether a prospective voter was educated enough to cast a ballot, but were often used to disqualify blacks, however literate, from voting. The story in question (quite likely apocryphal) involves a black preacher who was asked to read first English, then Hebrew, then Greek—all of which he successfully read. Then he was asked to read a laundry ticket covered in Chinese characters. The preacher responded: "It says, 'You're not going to vote today.'"

In both stories, the aggressor has prejudged the conclusion, so that the questioning is merely a pretense. You may well ask why people bother to go through phony exercises of this sort. The answer seems to be that people want to *appear* honest and fair even when they are behaving otherwise. They pretend to be acting for legitimate reasons rather than telling the truth: "I'm doing this because I want to and I can."

Prejudice is not entirely conscious, however, as suggested by common experience and backed up by research. You might be surprised to learn, for example, how simple it is to implant a bias in someone's mind, without that person's knowledge or even awareness. Let me give you three examples. In the early 1980s, psychologist Robert Zajonc conducted experiments in which he and his colleagues flashed images at people so briefly they were not even aware of the stimuli (that is, subliminally). They did not know that they had seen any images, let alone what the images showed. Nevertheless, when looking at pictures later in the experiment, they tended to prefer images they had seen subliminally over unfamiliar ones. This phenomenon, called "the mere exposure effect," has been seen many times in repeat experiments, leaving no doubt that, like it or not, human beings are clearly more comfortable with images (or people) that are familiar, as opposed to the unfamiliar or foreign.

In his book *The Righteous Mind*, Jonathan Haight cites a study in which a colleague hypnotized people and taught them to dislike a certain word. Then, while still in a trance, the subjects were told to forget they'd been instructed about the word. They were then returned to "normal" consciousness. The researchers then asked half the subjects to judge the morality of stories including the "bad" word and the other half to judge stories that were almost identical but lacked the "bad" word. As you might predict, the stories in the first set were judged more disgusting and morally reprehensible. Also, the character in one story was judged more harshly in the version that contained the "bad" word. Once again, people made value judgments without knowing how they got there.

Nevertheless—and here comes an important point—when pressed, most provided "explanations" for their conclusions. So powerful was the need to make sense of the unremembered instruction that their minds actually concocted pseudo-reasons to "explain" them.

Psychiatrists and other therapists see examples of these pseudo-explanations all the time. Sometimes the "explanation" is embraced by a person because it is less embarrassing or painful than the real reason—Freud called such "explanations" *rationalizations*. Sometimes the "explanation" derives from a person's general mood state. For example, when depressed, a woman may feel distant from her husband because "He never really loved me—nobody could." Yet that very same woman, when cheerful, may feel close to the husband, saying, "He is always so dependable; I love that I can count on him."

Similarly, neurophysiologists have found that when they stimulate certain brain regions in people who are conscious, the people respond in a way specific to the brain region involved. Yet the subjects of these experiments will manufacture reasons for that response. For example, when researchers stimulated a "humor center" in a young girl, she laughed. When asked why she was laughing, she said, "You guys look so funny, just standing around." Bottom line: The brain finds reasons to explain and justify however a person feels, though the explanations may have nothing to do with the real reason.

In the last study I want to mention, Harvard psychologist Dan Ariely asked a group of students to do two things: first to write down the last four digits of their Social Security numbers, and then to state the maximum amount of money they would be willing to pay for a list of luxury items. Surprisingly, the first number correlated with the second. In other words, someone whose Social Security number happened to end in 9550 was likely to offer more money for the items than someone with a number ending in 1550. This experiment and others like it have been repeated and reconfirmed: There is an "anchoring effect," such that one piece of information goes on to influence subsequent thoughts, feelings and behavior, often unconsciously and certainly irrationally. In Ariely's study, the students themselves were unaware of any correlation between the two unrelated numbers.

To sum up: Research shows the power of the familiar, the power of unconscious thoughts and feelings, and the power of anchoring—to influence conclusions, judgments, and behavior, even when it comes to relatively neutral things. In other words, we are—all of us are—prejudiced.

If such irrational prejudice exists in matters of no consequence, like people in made-up stories, how much more would we expect preconceptions to hold sway when the issue is highly emotional? For example, how fairly will we judge people whom we regard, rightly or wrongly, as threatening our jobs, competing with us for resources, or detracting from the value of our homes? How likely are we to provide sensible-sounding "reasons" for our prejudice? The real reason, of course, is usually simply that the people against whom we are prejudiced are just not like us—in skin color, language, religion, political leanings, sexual orientation, or some other feature we see as important.

Can prejudice be reversed? I believe so, though it is not easily done. An eighty-year-old client of mine, a highly intelligent and successful businessman, came in for a visit recently. He had been influenced by Haight's book to question his own prejudices. "Take gay marriage, for example," he said. "In Turkey, where I grew up, homosexuality was regarded as an abomination, so naturally I was opposed to gay marriage. But then I took the time to think about it clearly and asked myself: 'If two gay people want to get married, why should that affect me—or anyone else, for that matter? And if they've been together for thirty years and one of them gets sick, why shouldn't the other be able to visit him in the hospital?' And so forth." Soon my client found himself shifting his position on the issue.

This type of successful questioning of one's own gut feelings (which are often the basis for prejudice) provides hope that perhaps prejudice can be reversed at both the individual and societal levels. In the United States and other developed countries, such reversal appears to be happening in the case of gay marriage. Universal suffrage and reduced discrimination in the workplace also seem to be making gains around the world.

LET US SHIFT ATTENTION now to our second theme: Jane Austen's famous novel *Pride and Prejudice*, which, as its name implies, includes many instances of prejudice. The novel also helps us understand how prejudice predisposes us to the third, apparently unrelated topic in this chapter's title—sociopaths.

An early scene in the novel takes place at a country dance where Elizabeth, the brightest and most charming of the five Bennett daughters, overhears the handsome, rich, and haughty Mr. Darcy sneering at her looks. Unbeknownst to her (and him), he is actually attracted to her, but is prejudiced because of she is of lower social standing than himself. After overhearing his disparaging remarks, Elizabeth, as you might expect, develops a prejudice against Darcy. His pride! His unforgivable pride!

Subsequently, Elizabeth meets a handsome and charming soldier, George Wickham, who had grown up with Darcy. Wickham pours out to Elizabeth a story about how ill served he has been by Darcy's handling of his inheritance. He says Darcy had interfered with the elder Darcy's wish to see to it that Wickham was provided for. Perhaps because of her prejudice against Darcy, Elizabeth is ready to believe the whole tale as fact, even though she knows little about Wickham. Just as she is prejudiced *against* Darcy, she is now prejudiced *in favor of* Wickham. She likes him!—and, as Austen shrewdly observed, "How quick come the reasons for approving what we like!"

Wickham turns out to be a sociopath. He has previously attempted to seduce Darcy's younger sister, and he now proceeds to coldheartedly seduce and carry off *Elizabeth's* younger sister. His motive is money—to wangle a handsome sum from a family driven to buy silence and avoid the utter disgrace of a known seduction and elopement.

Sociopaths are people who lack conscience and are unable to empathize with others. Although we don't have a good understanding of how people become sociopaths, as a result of their deficits their life stories are often a litany of crimes, deceptions, damaged relationships (they are callously indifferent toward the feelings and well-being of others), and encounters with the law. Successful sociopaths can get away with their antisocial behaviors for a long time, in part because they are undeterred by scruple—all their intelligence is free to study how to mimic real emotions, turn on the charm, or spin a plausible yarn, no holds barred. Their ability to masquerade as normal is captured in the title of a classic book on the subject by Hervey Cleckley—*The Mask of Sanity*.

There is nothing like having tangled with a sociopath, or worse still, having been a victim of one, to learn their ways. A friend of mine who grew up with two sociopathic brothers has this to say about sociopaths: "They are expert at creating illusions—and will go to great lengths to do so—in order to ensnare their mark." Based on his experiences with his brothers and other sociopaths, he instinctively detects what he calls their "reptile eyes," which fail to register sincere emotion—though you have to be on the lookout to pick this up: the signal comes and goes in a blink. The effect is of a small feral animal that pops its head up to assess events, sees you watching, and ducks back out of sight. Also, the sociopathic smile is devoid of warmth. Many actually avoid smiling and expressing emotion, perhaps because they find that insincerity is easier to see through than a poker face, which can be mistaken for simple self-control.

In the next chapter, I will describe an unfortunate episode in my own life when I became entangled with a sociopath and his wily scheme.

Some years ago I reviewed Martha Stout's excellent book *The Sociopath Next Door* for *The Washington Post*. Stout's premise is that there are sociopaths all around us—even perhaps next door—who are capable of doing considerable harm, but are hard to spot. She sets out to help the reader do a better job of detection. Although most of Stout's observations were familiar to me, one struck me as novel and rather helpful: The sociopath often presents himself or herself as a victim and tells a sob story to elicit feelings in the mark—sympathy, compassion, or outrage—whatever helps further the sociopath's goals. That is what Wickham was doing with Elizabeth in *Pride and Prejudice,* and Austen with the eye of a brilliant clinician laid it all out for us.

> *Most people have prejudices against certain groups or ideas. It may be worth questioning your own prejudices.*
>
> *But be careful not to be prejudiced in favor of those who don't deserve your trust—such as sociopaths.*

Chapter 32

Lessons from a Scam

There's a sucker born every minute.

—OFTEN CREDITED TO P. T. BARNUM, BUT ACTUAL SOURCE UNCLEAR

The man who makes no mistakes does not usually
make anything.

—EDWARD JOHN PHELPS

Perhaps it is no coincidence that one of the experiences from which I learned the most was also one of my biggest mistakes: I got scammed. Perhaps my story will keep you from venturing into similar murky waters.

In 2008, the world watched a scam of epic proportions unfold in New York City, as the victims of Bernie Madoff lost millions of dollars—in some cases, everything they had. My heart went out to them. These people were by no means fools. Madoff's list of victims reads like a who's who for hedge funds, banks, foundations, and charities, along with a sprinkling of high-profile celebrities. Instead of wondering, How could they be so stupid? I say to myself, There but for the grace of God . . . because, indeed, I once fell into a similar trap.

Like Madoff's, "my" scam was a Ponzi scheme, named after Charles Ponzi, an early swindler who used this ploy. Essentially, Ponzi schemes promise unusually good returns, which they deliver (or appear to deliver) for a while. What the "investors" don't know is that no investment has been made. Any "payouts" they may receive come from their own capital or that of later "investors," who were lured in turn by the promise of large or consistent paper "yields." Usually the thing implodes when too many people want to withdraw their money or the supply of suckers runs out.

Most of us have heard that if something sounds too good to be true, it probably is. We know that. But sometimes a seductive little voice speaks up in the mind and says, "Except . . . except in this case." That voice can be fueled by many things, such as greed, need, an overripe imagination, or wishful thinking. What is seldom at work at the moment of signing is common sense, caution, or due diligence. In my case, all three were lacking.

Without going into detail as to how I got into the scam, let's start at that fateful moment when I endorsed a substantial check (enough to really hurt if I lost it) over to the scammer. That was the moment of no return.

What followed was a honeymoon period, as is often the case in a Ponzi scheme. I thought my money was being well tended. In this phase people are often eager to get in. When Madoff was flying high, for example, people vied with one another to join. They begged him to accept their money—an honor bestowed only on people with substantial wealth, power, or fame. As in all bad relationships, however, the honeymoon took a nasty turn. More people wanted out than in, there wasn't enough money to pay them off, and the jig was up.

I remember my feeling of disbelief when I learned that my money was gone, and the whole venture was a scam. Then came realization, anger (especially toward myself), and a slew of rhetorical questions: "How could I have been so stupid? How could I have done this to my family? How can I ever recover?" The final question, after I regrouped, was more to the point: "How can I get my money back?"

One element that had initially induced me to get involved with the con man was his alliance with a high-profile lawyer, who had a glossy brochure, a business card engraved on the finest stock, and a swanky downtown office. As I think of my naïveté in paying heed to these external trappings, embarrassment at my youthful self urges me to tell you that these incidents happened (luckily) many years ago. But though I was young, I was by no means helpless.

As a researcher, I knew that in order to develop a plan of action, you have to understand what and whom you are dealing with. To that end, a friend and I developed a history of the scam, which turned out to be so convoluted and tortuous that I'll spare you the details. We obtained information from other victims, though not all were willing to talk to us. In retrospect, some of the nontalkers had probably succeeded in getting their money out and were therefore, under the regulations that govern such schemes, susceptible to "clawback"—the requirement to pay back whatever you have drawn from your account so that the pool of salvaged money can be distributed evenly among the losers. But many others were helpful and appreciative.

Our project eventually led us to a lawyer, Marty, who had already agreed to represent a few of the victims, though he did not yet have a comprehensive picture of the scam. I liked Marty at once: firm, feisty, smart, and unintimidated by authority, he reminded me of my father. I knew immediately that he would be a great addition to our team. Marty, in turn, was delighted to have our written history, which put into perspective the miscellaneous bits and pieces of information that had come his way.

Marty and I agreed that I should meet with Edward, the lawyer in the swanky office who had allied himself with the con man, and sound him out—which I did. In the meeting, Edward got the con man on speakerphone and, after talking with him in my presence, promised to make me whole. But that was beyond his power to do, because the money was gone.

In the weeks that followed, Marty and I had further discussions with Edward and his lawyer, neither of whom ever acknowledged a smidgen of responsibility. We therefore filed a complaint against Edward, which went to arbitration. Edward's lawyer sought to portray me as an opportunist (like a supermarket slip-and-fall claimant) trying to take advantage of his client's innocent connection with a most unfortunate case. I countered with my side of the story, and soon—"soon" in a legal sense, meaning many months after the initial bad news—the matter was happily resolved. The picture of the scam we had developed and our strategy for recouping damages also provided a useful road map for the twenty-five other victims of the scam (also represented by Marty).

You may well wonder what became of Edward. He was imprisoned for scamming his own father out of a large sum of money. And the con man? A recidivist, he also went to jail—where he successfully scammed the daughter of his cell mate. When it came to sentencing, the judge, having reviewed his extensive history of fraudulent dealings, remarked that no place was safe from this man. If he were sent to a desert island, said the judge, he would scam the seagulls.

Here, Then, Are the Lessons I Learned from the Scam, the Gifts of This Rather Nasty Form of Adversity

1. Pick a really good spouse or life partner. My wife was an angel and didn't blame me—though she certainly had every right and reason to.

2. Pick some good friends: Ours came through for us in amazing ways. Some cousins offered us a large check as a gift.

I thanked them, but said that luckily we didn't need it. Another friend offered to have the crook "taken out," insisting that he knew people who would gladly do the job. I declined the offer. It was reassuring to realize that was not part of my nature.

3. Strange as it may seem, stories can be helpful. My accountant, for example, told me a story about how he had once dealt in precious gold coins, working with a particular dealer for many years. One day the dealer called and said that he had a buyer for the entire collection at an excellent price. My accountant turned over all his coins to the dealer, whereupon neither coins nor dealer were ever seen again. One of the most painful elements of having been scammed is the engulfing feeling of shame that one has of having been such a fool. Well, I knew my accountant to be smart and savvy, so the fact that he had made such an error irrationally but powerfully made me feel less stupid.

   In a later chapter (39), I discuss further the value of stories in overcoming adversity.

4. I learned once again that sometimes you can successfully fight back against adversity and injustice, using all the weapons at your disposal. In my case, they were the weapons of a psychiatrist, researcher, and writer. These skills must not have looked formidable to Edward and the con man, but I succeeded nonetheless, and so can you (if you have the misfortune of landing in such a mess in the first place).

   Also, I realized just how much law had rubbed off on me while growing up with my litigator father. On many occasions, Dad would say things like "We're not going to submit to such and such" or "Does he really think we're going to let him get away with that?" That feisty spirit had apparently entered me by osmosis. Maybe it would work for you too.

5. At some point during the process, I met an FBI agent who had been working on the scam, and told her my version of events. She was not, of course, at liberty to say much, but what she *did* say stuck with me.

    "Imagine that this whole business is like a house," she said, "and you are looking into just one window. Based on what you see through that window, you think you can reconstruct what is going on in the rest of the house. But you could be dead wrong."

    I have thought of her comment many times, because it can just as easily apply to anyone I meet, both in or out of my psychiatric office. People generally show one side of themselves, which may lead you to think you can complete the picture and have a comprehensive understanding of who they are—but you could be dead wrong. After years of experience, I have learned to make as few assumptions as possible about people.

6. At one point I said to my lawyer, Marty (who is by now an old friend), "How will I ever recover from this?" He said, "Don't be silly. People recover from all sorts of things much worse than this." And, of course, he was right, which is useful to remember. *It was only money at stake—not life.*

7. Thinking back on the scam, Marty said to me recently, "There was nothing unusual about it, except the way you fought back—and what a fight! It was like man bites dog."

8. Another benefit I hope I have acquired from the scam is a substantial immunity against being scammed again. So far, so

good. My hope in telling you this story is to pass some of that immunity on to you.

9. Perhaps I should give the last word to Marty. When the whole matter was over, he turned to me and said, "Sometimes the best lessons in life come from disasters that almost happen, but don't."

Before staking a large amount on a new venture, check it out with several independent qualified people. Watch out for any signs that something may be amiss, and don't discount any concerns you may have, no matter how small they may seem.

Finally, if you do have the misfortune to fall for a scam, fight back. With the help of others and a positive attitude, you may recoup some, if not all, of your losses.

Chapter 33

A Ghost from the Past

There must be ghosts all over the world. They must be as
countless as the grains of the sands, it seems to me.

—HENRIK IBSEN, *GHOSTS*

Human beings are not born once and for all on the day
their mothers give birth to them, but . . . life obliges them
over and over again to give birth to themselves.

—GABRIEL GARCÍA MÁRQUEZ

Sometimes as we happily go about our lives and all seems well,
we are startled by a ghost from the past. That's what happened to
me when I got routine blood work before a gastroscopy. My GI doctor at
the time was a tall, self-confident man with a large office lined with
certificates from top schools and programs, who usually dressed
sharply. But now, as I waited on the gurney for my procedure, he was
wearing scrubs. He greeted me in a hail-fellow-well-met kind of way and
told me we were good to go.

"And what about my blood work?" I asked him.

"The liver enzymes were a bit high and the hep C antibodies were positive," he said.

Hepatitis C!

"What's the significance of that?" I asked him.

"Let's discuss that after the procedure," he said.

I HAD AN INTRAVENOUS LINE running into my arm, the anesthesiologist had arrived, and before I had time to say more, I was out. I woke up to find my GI doctor showing me pictures he'd taken during the procedure.

"Look at this beauty," he said. "See how the camera captured the texture of the mucosa? And here, where the stomach curves toward the duodenum. Isn't that terrific?"

"Did you find anything abnormal?" I asked.

"No," he said, still gazing admiringly at the pictures.

"And what about the blood results?" I asked him, my mind as clear as the liquid still running into my vein, despite the lingering effects of the anesthetic. I'd gone out with this question ringing in my head, and it was ringing still.

"Your liver enzymes were high and hepatitis C antibodies were positive," he repeated.

"What's the implication of that?" I said.

"I haven't got time for a long story," he replied briskly.

"How about a short story then?" I asked angrily. It was obvious, even to someone just recovering from a procedure, that this doctor didn't want to take the time and trouble to communicate bad news to his patient.

He rattled off a few facts about hepatitis C, which he said progressed slowly but could ultimately be fatal. "Come and see me in my office," he said, "and we can discuss it further."

I never did see him again.

. . .

I REFLECTED ON THE NEWS. My liver enzymes had been mildly elevated for some time, but since these were early days in our knowledge of hepatitis C, my internist had not been alarmed; nor had he tested for hepatitis C. It was obviously time to bring in an expert.

Jay Hoofnagle, then a senior investigator in liver diseases at the National Institutes of Health, had an office in the same building as mine. I dropped in on him unannounced.

After a brief introduction (he knew who I was anyway), I blurted out, "I have hepatitis C." He seemed nonplussed and said nothing. "It's not the best diagnosis, is it?" I asked.

"It's not the worst," he said.

"How so?"

"Well," he said, "the viruses are just sitting out there in the cytoplasm of the liver cells." He spoke with animation, raising his hands in the air. "They're wriggling around there, just waiting for us to get them." And he wriggled his fingers as though they were viruses, exposed and ready to be zapped.

I thanked him and went on my way. Later that day he stopped by my office and apologized for not being more forthcoming. I had caught him by surprise, he said, but if I would like to make an appointment with him, it would be his pleasure to see me and treat me.

That was the start of a relationship with one of the few great doctors I have known as both patient and colleague. When you encounter a doctor who not only embodies old-world courtesy and empathy (what used to be called "a good bedside manner"), but also possesses the most up-to-date information and expertise, you are not just dealing with a good doctor but the *best*.

JAY AND I watched my liver enzymes over time. I suspected that I had become infected via the blood transfusion I received after being stabbed in South Africa. That was confirmed when the virus turned out to be of a type essentially found only in South Africa. A liver biopsy showed minimal inflammation. So although I'd been infected for twenty-four years, the viruses had not done much damage to my liver. Luckily, hep C usually moves slowly. Nevertheless, we could not rely on that to continue.

The best treatment at the time was interferon, injected under the skin three times a week, plus an antiviral drug, which I resisted. For one thing, the combination did not always work. For another, in some people, interferon causes profound depression, so serious that they are unable to tolerate the treatment. That scared me, because I needed to stay functional. At a certain point, however, Jay said we should go for it. "You don't want to be dealing with this as an old man," he said. "Rather get over it now." That made sense.

I scheduled no patients for the day after my first interferon shot, because I didn't know how it would affect me. But to my surprise, I felt quite well, so the next day, when the wife of a patient called, I was able to take the call and listen. She told me of a crisis with her husband, whom I had been treating for alcoholism. He had suffered a relapse and gone to bed, and now she was unable to rouse him. I recommended that she call 911 and take him to the emergency room, but she demurred. "The neighbors would see the ambulance and ask questions," she said. "It would be *so* embarrassing."

How about if I come over? I suggested—something I could not normally have offered, except that today my schedule was empty. She thought that was a great idea, so I set out for the house.

When I got there, my patient was beginning to stir, and since house calls are so unusual these days, he was embarrassed to find his doctor in his bedroom—but it was a good thing I was there. It took the two of us, his wife and me, to bundle him into their SUV and off to the ER—the first step in a lasting rehabilitation.

My patient and his wife were grateful to me for coming out to help. What they did not know at the time, however, was how grateful I was to *them.* That was my first day postinterferon, and I had feared that I would be useless. In helping this delightful couple, I had demonstrated to myself that I could function quite well on interferon. It gave me hope that the rest of the year might pass without a hitch, which, in fact, it did. The viruses proved to be as vulnerable as Jay Hoofnagle's wriggling fingers had suggested. I didn't miss a day of work, and though the people close to me said I was a bit crabby, my patients did not appear to notice any change.

I STILL VISIT Jay Hoofnagle at the NIH from time to time, as much for the pleasure of his company as any other reason. Sometimes his colleagues ask for samples of my blood, to see whether they can learn what it is about my particular T cells that helped me eliminate the virus. I always tell them to take as much as they want.

Once in a while, we are visited by ghosts from our past.

Should a ghost visit you, treat it as a challenge and tackle it with all the resources you can muster. As with all adventures, be open to learning, and pick the right friends, fellows (and doctors) to see you through the journey.

Chapter 34

Don't Hold On to Grudges

Before you embark on a journey of revenge, dig two graves.

—CONFUCIUS

Grudges are like a fire in the heart.

—MAHARISHI MAHESH YOGI

was thinking recently of Sara, a former patient of mine, who used to maintain a "grudge list." Every time she felt that somebody had slighted or harmed her in any way, she would make a careful note of it. As a result, her grudge list kept getting longer over time. As I thought about Sara, I wondered who was on *my* grudge list. As you now know, I have sustained some injuries—as anyone would who has lived a certain number of years. But even the idea of taking inventory of those hurts feels creepy. It is against my nature—and I don't recommend it to others. For as I contemplated Sara and her grudge list, I felt grateful. I have no grudge list. What a relief!

Though I am no anthropologist, I have seen grudges play out in different ways in different societies I have known. They seem to have some use in regulating social behavior. For example, the tribal Tswanas, among whom I worked, believed that grudges could bring down the wrath of ancestral spirits against the grudgee, who might, as a consequence, develop an illness or some other misfortune. The fear of incurring a lethal grudge kept people in line and prevented misbehavior.

One society famous for grudges and retribution is organized crime. As we all know from the *Godfather* movies, it is a small step from a grudge to revenge, which often results in the spilling of blood. Revenge brings retaliation—more shooting and more blood—resulting in an ongoing vendetta between the feuding parties. Confucius understood the dangers of revenge: "dig two graves" indeed.

In the Jewish community of Johannesburg, grudges took on a special form and were given a special name—*faribels*. Such *faribels* usually arose as a result of social slights. If someone didn't invite you to his daughter's wedding, you would register a *faribel* and hold on to it till you could even the score—for example, at *your* daughter's wedding. Withholding invitations may not be the stuff of great moviemaking. It's hardly a shoot-out. But some found a certain comfort in the knowledge that as the band was playing "Hava Nagila" and your grudgee was sitting alone at home, the pain of ostracism would be sharper than a serpent's tooth.

So it seems as though, at the level of society, fear of incurring a grudge gives people an incentive to act friendly and restrain aggression. What effects, however, do grudges have on the grudge bearer? Several bad effects and nothing good, as best I can tell.

At a cognitive level, bearing grudges—or feeling resentment—means adopting the role of a victim, which is disempowering. That's why I bridled at the idea of taking inventory of my injuries. Being a victim just doesn't seem like a useful path to take. It's far better, in my view, to say, "Okay, these bad things happened. Now what can I do about it? And if there's nothing I can do, how soon can I let it go?"

From an emotional point of view, bearing a grudge nurtures a particular type of simmering anger. It is usually easy to detect when someone is angry at you—we are programmed to have that skill. So if you are walking around the world angry, others know it, and they will respond with fear, avoidance, or anger in return—all responses that do you no good. In my experience, kindly and generous people often (though not always) receive kindness even from strangers. Conversely, angry people often find their anger reflected back at them.

One aspect of bearing grudges that fascinates me as a physician and psychiatrist is that chronic anger can harm you physically. Researchers have found that hostility is associated with cardiovascular disease, the single biggest killer in developed countries. The widely used Minnesota Multiphasic Personality Inventory (MMPI) has a subscale that measures hostility, a word that technically refers not only to a tendency to get angry but also to a cynical mistrust of others and a tendency to attribute hostile motivations to them. Grudge bearers tend to look for occasions to feel slighted, so that they can add to their collection. They will take personally a slight that someone else might disregard. For example: Someone else may say, "He didn't invite me to the wedding because numbers are limited and we're not that close." The grudge bearer, however, is more apt to say, "He deliberately excluded me out of spite," or, "I'm just not important enough to make the list." Those kinds of thoughts are associated with unhappiness, stress, and ill health. They can take years off your life.

In one very convincing study, researchers at Duke University administered the MMPI to students at the University of North Carolina (UNC) medical and law schools. Twenty-five years later, for both physicians and lawyers, hostility scores measured during their student years strongly predicted whether they'd be dead or alive. Some cardiologists have suggested that being hostile may be as bad for your cardiac health as smoking or eating fatty foods. I can certainly think of several angry people in my practice over the years who have ended up with stents and bypass surgery.

All in all, regardless of how you feel about the morality of bearing grudges, it is probably wise to avoid them, if only for your health.

As quoted above, Maharishi referred to grudges as "a fire in the heart." I have always thought of them as an acid that corrodes the vessel that contains it.

> *Grudges probably harm those who harbor them more than those at whom they are directed. So if only for your own sake, avoid registering grudges, and if you have a grudge list, tear it up!*

Chapter 35

Hold On to Dreams

Cherish your visions and your dreams as they
are the children of your soul, the blueprints of
your ultimate achievements.

—NAPOLEON HILL

All achievements, all earned riches, have their
beginning in an idea.

—NAPOLEON HILL

In order to accomplish any long-term goal, it is useful and perhaps
necessary to have a dream—a dream as distinct from just an idea.
Both are necessary but, as is apparent in the two quotes above by the
famous motivational writer Napoleon Hill, they have a different quality
to them. An idea dwells in the cognitive, rational part of the mind. It
may be part of a dream, but a dream is also infused with passion, which
gives it additional power. As writer Mary Wollstonecraft explained,
"When we feel deeply, we reason profoundly." When these two types of
mental processes work together—cognition and emotion—you have

the basis for a dream: something that grabs you with both hands, rivets you intellectually, emotionally, and physically, and sustains your focus over time.

J. K. Rowling, for example, describes how when she first conceived the idea of Harry Potter, she felt excitement tingling throughout her body—an indication to her that she had hit upon an important creative idea, not just another ho-hum notion. When I first recognized the syndrome of seasonal affective disorder, my body registered that same type of excitement. I was reading through questionnaire responses from person after person, telling similar stories of how they became depressed in fall and winter, and felt better in spring and summer. And as I read, I realized that we had stumbled on a new syndrome with a potentially new type of treatment. I literally shivered with excitement.

A dream in the sense of a vision resembles a regular dream or daydream in that it involves a shift in consciousness and gives access to realms of mind not always accessible in a waking state.

The dreams about which I am writing here could refer to any important goal. It could be personal—your dream of getting married or moving to a new country, becoming a concert violinist, a major-league baseball player, an engineer, or an architect. Or you could frame the very same dream in terms of its impact on the world, such as delighting people with your music or athletic prowess, bringing clean water to a village, building a school, or making the world a better place in some special way. Whatever the goal, personal or transpersonal, the elements of how to attain it are the same: Recognize your own unique and authentic dream, take it seriously (even if others don't), and sustain it over time—even if it morphs, as dreams often do. As we grow and mature, so do our dreams.

All of us, I believe, have dreams: small or big, realistic or unrealistic. Aside from their associated goals, the dreams themselves are a source of pleasure, as they enlarge our lives and expand our sense of the impact we can have on the world.

So, how does the dreamer meet adversity? Dreams are often consuming, draining us of our time and energy. They can deprive us of ordinary pleasures and make us less available to others. They can be costly to our loved ones too, who may find us distracted and inattentive because we are so preoccupied. (If you are aware of this cost, you can take measures to mitigate it—which I encourage you to do for the sake of your loved ones.) Dreams often involve sacrifice, and their success is by no means guaranteed. Yet I heartily subscribe to them, based on both personal experience and my work with patients. Dreams sustain us.

Of course, in order for a dream to come true, it must have some basis in reality. I have had lots of dreams in my life. Some were idle and unrealistic, while others . . . well, they seemed possible. When I was very young, I told my mother I wanted to find a cure for cancer. It wasn't really my dream. I had borrowed it from a friend whose father was a doctor, and I thought it sounded rather grand. I overheard my mother telling her friend on the beach about this ambition, and the friend laughed. "How cute," she said. I didn't like being patronized, but it did me no harm, perhaps because it wasn't my dream. The experience did teach me, though, not to laugh at other people's dreams.

As I reached my teens, my dreams coalesced around understanding the human mind, but it wasn't clear what form that might take. Research? Writing novels? Writing about the mind more directly? It is instructive, perhaps, that I received very little encouragement, yet became a psychiatrist and writer nonetheless. It shows the power of dreams—that my parents were unable to interfere with them, though goodness knows they tried. Loathsome as the idea of psychiatry was to them, being a writer was even worse. When they discussed this latter ambition with a neighbor who ran a successful dress shop, she snorted: "From this you can make a living?"

"Exactly!" cried my parents. "Case closed!"

My father told me about the many doctors who had gone on to become writers *after* completing their medical training (it was an impressive list). I felt as if I were being handled, which I was. But the handling worked—not so much because it was expertly done, because it was not. Rather, it worked because of two forces maneuvering within me. First, I was genuinely interested in the mind and the brain, but second—equally important—I lacked the confidence that I could write anything of value. Which, I realize now, was at that time accurate. I was only sixteen, after all. I had no medical or literary training, not to mention experiences worth writing about. Most important, perhaps, I lacked the ability to occupy in a sustained way the inner world that the writer needs to inhabit.

As the years passed, I did acquire experiences worth recording, such as my role in describing SAD and developing light therapy; that became the basis for *Winter Blues*, and other books followed. One of these, a sprawling tome called *The Emotional Revolution*, was exciting to me because of its subject matter—the entire emerging science of emotions. But the subject was too diffuse and encyclopedic for most readers. I remember discussing the project with the British editor of a previous book of mine. "There is a saying," I told her, "that the fox has many tricks, but the porcupine has one big trick. I want this new book to be like a fox, with many tricks that show you how to improve your emotional life."

"Sometimes," she replied very sweetly, "it's easier to sell a book with one big trick."

Her words were prophetic. *The Emotional Revolution* did not do well commercially. In fact, when Leora and I reviewed how many hours I had spent writing it, we realized that my hourly compensation had been not much more than the minimum wage. "That's it!" Leora said. "We just can't afford for you to write any more books." And I agreed—for some years, at least.

But then something strange happened, as it often does with books: Some mental health professionals loved the *The Emotional Revolution*, and one person felt it had changed her life. She referred a friend to me, who referred another friend, and so it went. This chain of referrals led me to my next passion—Transcendental Meditation (TM).

Not only did I become intellectually excited about TM's potential to help many people in our stressed-out, war-torn world, but I had a powerful experience of its effects on myself. Before I started meditating, my overactive "monkey mind" had made it near impossible for me to sit down alone in a quiet place and delve into my thoughts—which is crucial for writing anything of depth and substance. In addition, ideas came to me during meditation—unexpected phrases, memories of clever things other people had said and curious things they had done. I felt as though TM had given me the final set of tools to make me a writer: the capacity for solitude, access to my unconscious creative wellsprings, and a sustained capacity to produce. I was ready now to follow the recommendation of my British editor—to write a porcupine of a book, a book with one big trick. That book, appropriately, turned out to be *Transcendence: Healing and Transformation Through Transcendental Meditation.*

That brings us to the present. All my life, like most people, I have gathered lessons along the way, embedded in stories that go with them. Only now, though, do I have the wherewithal to sort them out and write them in a way that might help anyone besides myself. Yet I held on to my dream. I waited. I persisted. I tried new things, and I grew—and in time, some of my dreams have been realized.

I hope my journey may help those who despair about their potential to fulfill their own dreams, which may seem too difficult or too far in the future. The long view is especially important nowadays, as we often read about people who seem to fulfill their dreams overnight. They go from building computers or writing software in their parents' garages to becoming billionaires in their twenties. These fabulous stories are inspiring, but they are the exception, not the rule. For some of us, the journey from the inception of a dream to its fulfillment is a matter of decades, not years.

I am by no means suggesting that you delay your journey. Start today. Dream boldly and plentifully. The world will show you what is and is not feasible—and that will probably change over time, as the world changes and you develop new strengths and skills. There is usually no need to rush; do not truncate the scope of your vision before giving yourself a chance to grow to your full potential.

And remember, new and even larger dreams may come along—dreams that you have yet to dream. A poet can become an artist; a computer whiz a philanthropist; an actor the president. Such transformations are occurring all the time. I can't wait to see what new dreams may come my way.

Also, we are lucky to be living in the twenty-first century, when improvements in medical care have given us significantly more years in which to fulfill our dreams. Use the extra years to create something huge and wonderful—like the Golden Gate Bridge—that can span the course of a lifetime.

> *Take your dreams seriously even if others don't.*
>
> *Hold on to them firmly, if necessary over decades, and let them grow.*
>
> *And then, with hard work and good fortune, all your dreams can come true.*

Chapter 36

Taking Responsibility

Lessons from Dad and from Life

Once the rockets are up, who cares where they come down?
That's not my department.
—WERNHER VON BRAUN, FORMER NAZI, U.S. ROCKET SPECIALIST
  (AS RELAYED BY TOM LEHRER)

When you think everything is someone else's fault,
you will suffer a lot.
—THE DALAI LAMA

On one occasion, a patient had to bring along her two children, a six-year-old girl and the child's younger brother, who found their way from my waiting room into a neighbor's garden. Alas, the garden had a very tempting pond, and the day was hot. My neighbor called me, enraged, to say that the children were not only at risk themselves but (and this seemed to bother her as much or more) were putting *her* at risk for liability.

After the children were summoned indoors by their mother, the first words spoken came from the boy. "*She* suggested it! It was *her* idea!" he blurted out. Clearly afraid he'd be punished for their escapade, he preemptively sought to shift the blame.

His behavior, in fact, was not unlike that of my angry neighbor. To me, the scenario seemed to represent a common dynamic in our culture—the avoidance of blame at all costs. How different it would have felt if the neighbor had said only that she was concerned that the children were in danger, or if the children had said, "We're sorry we worried you."

In my childhood home, when my sisters and I were growing up, personal responsibility was emphasized at every turn. My lawyer father turned the dinner table into a courtroom, with himself in the judge's seat. For example, confronted by shards of glass, he might say:

"What happened to the glass?"

"It broke."

"Things don't break; people break them. Who broke it?"

And then, of course, there was the matter of cleaning up the mess. I thought of that recently when riding in the first-class coach of an upscale train that travels the northeast corridor of the United States. A businessman had set up office at the bulkhead and was talking loudly on his cell phone. He was making predictions about the forthcoming election, naming all the people and entities who had called him for his opinions, both on and off the air, and describing how this could all be "maximally monetized." In the middle of the conversation, he knocked over a glass, which broke into daggerlike shards, some of which lay on the floor pointing directly upward. He went right on talking as a woman with thin-soled shoes hurried by, almost treading on one of the daggers. He showed no interest in the matter, and no responsibility for drawing the staff's attention to the hazard (which I proceeded to do).

But back to the dinner-table courtroom. One of us three kids might complain that another had hit him or her, to which Dad would respond to the complainant, "Oh, and what did you do to provoke the attack?"

Or one of us might tell a story about how we had been driving and had the right of way, when another driver went against the light and almost clipped our car. Dad would retort, "Never mind who has the right of way. It will do you little good to have that written on your tombstone." His message was: Don't focus on what the other person is doing—focus on what *you* are doing. Your safety is the priority, and you are responsible for taking care of it.

One day Dad came home and told me about a man he was representing in a divorce case. Highly principled, in divorce cases he would always try to understand the nature of the conflict and explore the possibility of a reconciliation before proceeding legally.

"My client—I'll call him Cal—is filing for divorce for the third time," Dad told me. "I asked him what went wrong with the first marriage.

"'She was a nasty piece of work,' he responded.

"'And the second marriage?'

"'Even worse.'

"'And the current marriage?'

"'She's the worst of the bunch.'

"Now think about it," Dad said to me. "One nasty piece of work—okay, bad luck. Two nasty pieces, really bad luck—maybe. But three nasty pieces? You have to begin to question your judgment." Dad took the case without attempting to analyze his client's psychological problems. Shrewd as he was in the workings of the human mind, his arts were those of a lawyer, not a therapist.

In many ways, the lawyer's goals are opposite those of the therapist. The lawyer seeks to minimize the client's responsibility in the mind of client, judge, and jury. "What would you say to someone who came into your office and told you he was guilty?" I asked him once.

"I'd encourage him to take his time," Dad said, "and review what happened step by step. Maybe he's taking too much responsibility for what happened. Maybe there were mitigating factors, like self-defense. I'd try to find an angle to help him soften his stance."

And indeed, Dad worked hard to exonerate his clients, rich or poor, and became known as a fighter. (He had, in fact, been a boxer in his younger days.) One impoverished man he represented was accused of raping a woman. My father, having probed the details of the case, asked the judge whether he might approach the bench to make a highly unusual request. The request was granted. My father then instructed his client to drop his trousers. An audible gasp echoed through the courtroom as the exercise revealed that the accused had no penis! Case dismissed!

Many people enter psychotherapy for problems they see as the result of repeated bad luck or the misbehavior of others. Such chronic failure to take responsibility leaves people feeling like victims of fate rather than architects of their own destiny, which is not an empowering frame of mind. Why do they think this way? Because it is painful to admit errors and shortcomings. It is generally far more painful, however, to suffer the consequences of these deficiencies as they play out over time. That's what happens to people who habitually fail to take responsibility for their actions.

Avoidance of responsibility and blame shows up often in relationships. One common example: A wife suspects her husband of having an affair (or the other way around). The suspicious party raises the question, and the spouse denies it out of hand. Unsatisfied, she or he then finds a way to surveil the partner's computer and, sure enough, finds flirtatious e-mails, suggestive of an affair, but not definitive proof. The aggrieved party then confronts the partner with "the evidence."

What happens next? Here are some possible responses: (1) "This is just harmless flirtation; anyone should realize that." (2) "How dare you invade my privacy!" (3) "Although I am not having an actual physical affair with this person, I shouldn't be engaging in an exchange of flirtatious e-mails. I'm sorry to have been deceptive and caused you distress."

(4) "I have indeed been having an affair. I'm sorry on many levels, and I'd like to work on getting our marriage back on track."

In my experience, the first two responses are by far the most common. Why? Of course, there are legal and financial implications to admitting wrongdoing. But over and above these, it's unpleasant to take the rap for a major infraction. By denying the matter, people hope to kick the can farther down the road, and perhaps things will somehow get better by themselves. Although this hope sometimes comes true, more often the breach of trust deepens over time, wearing away the fabric of the relationship.

In the area of infidelity, the most egregious repudiation of responsibility I have ever encountered comes from—you guessed it—the annals of my father's legal tales. One of my father's clients walked in to find his wife in bed with another man, whereupon the lover, infuriated at being interrupted, jumped out of bed and punched the poor husband in the nose!

People may learn how to shirk responsibility at a young age, and the trait then continues through adolescence and into adulthood. In many instances, parents have not been diligent enough to catch the problem early and help their children correct it while they are still young (when it is easier). Josh, who sees many people with drug problems, has pointed out to me how often drugs compound problems with taking responsibility, and I agree. The two go together: Habitual drug users often insist on feeling good quickly and often. Over time, the personality deteriorates as the drugs train the brain to expect quick rewards following a drink, pill, snort, or needle. Somewhere down the line, usually sooner rather than later, the question of responsibility simply becomes irrelevant.

The path to recovery, if it occurs, is slow. First the drugs have to go; then a process of rehabilitation follows. A key part of rehabilitation is taking responsibility. In fact, the twelve steps of Alcoholics Anonymous and similar programs for drug, food, and sex addicts include taking inventory of your character defects; making amends to those you have hurt; continually surveying your ongoing behavior; and, when you are wrong, admitting it promptly. One of the steps also points out the value of prayer and meditation. I will discuss meditation as a tool to help people cope with drug abuse and impulsivity in chapter 40.

You don't have to be a therapist or a cuckolded spouse in order to encounter blame avoidance. It's everywhere. I have begun to play a little game with myself—to detect the many maneuvers people employ to avoid responsibility in everyday life. How often, for example, does the waiter who delivers the wrong order say, "They messed up in the kitchen," instead of, "Sorry for the mistake; I'll correct it at once." How often does a colleague who is late for lunch say, "The highway was a parking lot," instead of, "I'm so sorry; I left my office late"? It's an enjoyable game to play, in part because it makes blame avoidance by others less irritating. Every now and then, however, someone does say, "I'm sorry. I messed up. Please forgive me." How refreshing that is!

Taking responsibility is vital in business. For some years I was CEO of a small clinical-trials company, and as such, the ultimate responsibility for our results rested with me. Even though I always tried to do an excellent job, I remember at least one instance when I failed: We recruited too few subjects for a study, and the data were substandard. To make matters worse, the study sponsor was a major client. Needless to say, they didn't come knocking on our door for quite a while, until a friend recommended they give us another try.

The leader of the new study took me out on the balcony of the hotel at a professional meeting and interrogated me about the earlier study. I took it on the chin, acknowledged our underperformance, and asked him to give us another chance. I assured him that I would supervise the study in person. He must have been persuaded, because we got the job, and performed well. Had I made excuses about our prior performance, I doubt there would have been such a happy outcome. I learned valuable lessons from being responsible for running my own business—as well as from clients, who are highly successful businessmen and -women: Everybody makes mistakes—mistakes are our best teachers, so don't waste them. Acknowledge them, learn from them, and become more competent because of them.

But acknowledging responsibility in business can be tricky, because it raises the specter of liability—a major concern in the medical field. The liability wars have resulted in an atmosphere in which physicians and other health care personnel are reluctant to apologize for anything—often forbidden, in fact. To a patient who has been treated rudely or incompetently, such a blank wall adds insult to injury. It could even precipitate a complaint or lawsuit when a simple, sincere apology might have settled the matter.

An extraordinary story along these lines comes from a friend who was researching a magazine article about what happens when doctors make mistakes. An eminent, much-loved pediatrician told her this story: A child in his practice developed meningitis, but it was atypical and he missed the diagnosis until it was too late—and the child was profoundly brain damaged. As you can imagine, telling the parents was one of the worst moments of the doctor's life.

"What happened?" my friend asked.

He answered, "We wept together."

Not all parents would be so forgiving, but his obviously heartfelt response to their child's tragedy made him human in the parents' eyes and allowed them to share their grief with him, rather than seeing him as the enemy.

The last story I will tell you about taking responsibility concerns Elaine, a friend of many years, who was an acknowledged expert in her field of mental health. I wanted to interview Elaine for an earlier book, but had trouble connecting with her, and when I did, she always seemed short and irritable. I confronted her gently over the phone, and told her that even strangers had granted me interviews (which she had avoided doing), and they had been gracious about it. Her behavior was an anomaly.

To my very pleasant surprise, Elaine immediately acknowledged that she had been "off" and invited me to lunch. When we met, she told me how much she appreciated our friendship and offered to help with my book in any way she could. She was as good as her word, and I was glad to include her contributions. There is a sad end to this story. A few years after our minor conflict, Elaine developed a serious illness and died within a year of being diagnosed. We talked and visited often during that year, and the warmth we had always felt for each other was stronger than ever.

By acknowledging her brusque behavior and going out of her way to make amends, Elaine not only salvaged our friendship, she strengthened it. She left me with many fond memories, as well as a model for how to take responsibility for an injured relationship and mend it.

Take responsibility for your actions, including your errors and oversights. Apologize and make amends when appropriate. These practices are conducive to success and to a sense that you are in control of your life, not a victim of fate.

Chapter 37

Reciprocity in Relationships

Treat others as you would like them to treat you.

Do not treat others as you would not like them to treat you.

—THE GOLDEN RULE OR ETHIC OF RECIPROCITY

  (CAN BE FOUND IN SOME FORM IN MANY RELIGIONS)

Tit for tat: Blow for blow; retaliation in kind.

—*WEBSTER'S* DICTIONARY

One evening Leora and I went out for a casual dinner in one of those restaurants where the tables are rather close. To make matters worse, the acoustics were so poor that sound carried with an efficiency better suited to an opera house.

Not far from us sat another couple, somewhat younger than us, who were having an obvious first-date conversation. "Where did you go to school? What is your zodiac sign?" And so on. But the conversation soon devolved into a monologue, with him talking and her listening. He went on and on and on about his business accomplishments, his future plans, office politics and how he planned to handle it, his interests, his hobbies, his pets. . . . And she smiled . . . and smiled. It looked like an attempt at a Nancy Reagan smile (the one she used to hold when her husband was talking in public), but less adoring and more effortful. Her discomfort grew visibly as the dinner wore on.

I kept wanting to go over and say to him, "Why don't you ask her something about herself—anything?" Leora said she wanted to ask *her* why she was bothering to please such a clod—though neither of us did so, of course. I realize that this story might seem like a trivial example of the subject at hand—the importance of reciprocity in relationships— but I tell it because the dynamic was so clear, so pure, so detached from the messiness of actual relationships that its essence is easy to see: Here, right from the start of a possible relationship, one person was making it clear whose life mattered and whose did not. Though I have no way to follow up, I would be surprised if the couple got to a second date.

You don't need to be a psychiatrist to realize that the man in the restaurant has problems with reciprocity, which will cause problems in his relationships. Apparently nobody has ever taught him that in a conversation between two people, both should have a chance to speak; or, more fundamentally, that both have something to contribute. Everyone has the need (and right) to be listened to, not just talked at.

Although the behavior of the man in the restaurant was extreme, the basic dynamic is quite common—perhaps as a result of changes in parenting style. Parents these days seem so eager to foster their children's ability to express themselves, and are so intrigued by whatever their children have to say, that they are perhaps forgetting to foster the other half of the equation—the art of listening, along with other aspects of the golden rule.

The golden rule, as defined at the head of this chapter, represents an ideal worth striving for. To understand reciprocity in relationships, however, we have to acknowledge a second principle, which is encapsulated by the succinct expression "tit for tat." The expression goes back at least as far as the fifteen hundreds, but the principle it represents is, of course, far older. People tend to reward good behavior by others and punish bad behavior—as do members of several other species, including monkeys, birds, fish, and even vampire bats! These behaviors, known to biologists as reciprocal altruism, involve several principles, one of which is the ability to detect cheaters—those who defect from the principle of tit for tat.

In computer models that repeatedly play against each other in recurring scenarios in which they can either cooperate or defect, a simple model, appropriately called "Tit for Tat," proves to be highly effective. This model resembles reciprocal altruism in animals: It starts by cooperating and then does whatever the opposing program does—rewards cooperation and punishes defection. You could consider it to be forgiving, since it will cooperate immediately after the opposing program cooperates. In that regard, it doesn't "hold grudges." An even more forgiving program, appropriately named "Tit for Tat with Forgiveness," which occasionally refrains from punishing its opponent's defection, may be superior in certain situations. Just as in life, it sometimes pays to err on the forgiving side, especially in dealing with close friends and family.

LET ME SHARE WITH YOU two situations where reciprocity arose as an issue in my own life—one in the professional and one in the personal domain.

When I started my clinical-trials business, I was determined not only to do first-rate work but also to create an atmosphere where people felt fairly treated and appreciated. I made up my mind that if it was necessary to lay people off, they would get plenty of advance notice, as well as help finding another job.

One young man, Dean, was a fine research coordinator. We treated him well and he seemed happy in the job. Imagine my surprise when I found out he had been looking for other work for some time, having acquired references from a previous employer. Only once his new posi-

tion was firmly in place did he tell us that he was leaving. Losing Dean
was a blow to a small company like ours, where every person counts and
it takes months to recruit and train someone new. It also struck me as
such an unnecessary strategy on his part. Had he only told us he wanted
to move on, we would gladly have worked with him to find a solution
that suited us all.

Since this was the second time such an event had occurred in the
organization, I realized I needed to change its culture. In our group
meetings, I introduced the staff to the concept of reciprocity in
relationships—at work as at home. Just as management would not ter-
minate employees abruptly and without fair warning, so we expected
the same from them. If we were unhappy with their work, we would let
them know and give them a chance to do better. Likewise, if they were
unhappy with us, *we* wanted to know, and we promised not to hold it
against them if they wanted to find another job. Indeed, we would help
them: We would give the best possible evaluations, make the transition
pleasant, and provide future recommendations as needed. After we
implemented this intervention, we never had another worker leave sur-
reptitiously. Of course, we kept our end of the bargain, too.

A year or two after he left our organization, Dean called to ask
whether I would recommend him for a new position.

"Does your current employer know you are looking?" I asked him.

"No," he said. I asked him why not.

"It's a bit of a sticky situation here," he replied. "So I'm going to have
to finesse things."

I declined to provide the recommendation (one of the few times in
more than thirty years that I have ever done so). He was shocked. I explained to him that I did not think he had reciprocated our decency
and forthrightness in our dealings with him and that I would not participate in his doing the same to someone else. And that is the last time
we ever spoke.

In defense of Dean, I should say that in many work environments, people are laid off at short notice without cause, sometimes quite harshly. However, it should have been obvious to Dean that our small business was not such an organization.

NOW FOR AN EXAMPLE in the personal domain: I remember once, when Josh was in college, that he agreed to help me do some full-time library research for a book I was writing on St. John's wort. He worked hard and dug up some terrific references, but at the end of the first week he told me his cousin was coming to visit, so he'd have to take the next week off.

I was disappointed and concerned about meeting my deadline. I told Josh that his work was important to me, that I needed him, and that he had made a commitment. I appealed to his decency and his recognition that relationships should be reciprocal. No further discussion was needed. Josh subsequently told me that he had learned a valuable lesson from that experience—the need to uphold his end of a deal.

In my work as a psychiatrist I have encountered many people, of widely varying ages, who seem never to have thought about the need for commitments and reciprocity. Like the man on the first date, they are insensitive to the needs of others. That deficit is bad news for them, and also for the important people in their lives. In my experience, if the golden rule (do unto others) has not been instilled in people during their early years, it is difficult to do so later, because it involves several skills that are best learned early—notably empathy, responsibility, and kindness, especially to those who have been kind to them. Parents may think that they are serving their children well by encouraging them to focus largely on getting their own needs met, and by making life comfortable and easy for them. But they would do well to ask: What kind of adults will they grow up to be if they are not taught the art of reciprocity when they are young? They may learn from life, but I imagine a hard road ahead. As adults, how will these people care for those who love them—including the very parents who gave them everything and asked for nothing in return?

That's one reason it's so important for parents to teach their children empathy, to ask, "How do you think he or she will feel if you say or do that?" Likewise, children can be taught to ask one another—and even adults—"How was *your* day?" or, "I heard you were sick. How are you feeling?" And to listen to the answer!

These will be especially important lessons as the world becomes a more difficult home for humanity—hotter, stormier, more crowded, less secure. If ever there were a good time for restoring the centrality of the golden rule, it is now. If parents are clear with their children about the need to reach out to others and the value of fairness, reciprocity, and generosity, they may save both their children and themselves a lot of heartache down the line.

> *Teach your children the importance of reciprocity at an early age—in conversation, collaboration, and materially. You will be helping them in the long run, and, person by person, you will be making the world a better place.*

Chapter 38

Learning Something from Everyone

Who is wise? The one who learns something
from every person.

—TALMUD

M y father always used to say, "Free advice is worth the money you
pay for it." I disagree, though many people don't value what they
don't pay for. In my view, that is a big mistake. Some of my most valuable lessons, as you know from reading this book, have cost me nothing.
If we are vigilant, life presents us with free lessons almost every day.
Having developed this approach in my own life, I tried to encourage my
son to adopt the same attitude. I always sought out opportunities for
Josh to learn from people with differing perspectives, who deliver their
lessons in different voices and different ways. And that, in itself, has
been a lesson for me.

. . .

I FIRST BECAME AWARE of how much Josh could learn from others after he returned from a two-week Boy Scout camp. One evening after dinner he and I were loading the dishwasher when he began to clean the countertop as well. I was surprised, as veteran parents can imagine, and Josh noticed. He then explained that the scoutmaster had told the troop that it was important not to always wait for instructions. Instead, a good scout should look around and observe for himself what needs to be done, then do it. What a gift that was, not only to Josh but also to Leora and me.

I learned many things from this experience. First, here was excellent advice that had come from someone else. Second, I would most likely not have thought to give the advice so simply and effectively. Finally, even if I had, I doubt Josh would have listened as well to me. When I asked Josh about this recently—he is now a psychiatrist himself—he explained, "Your parents are always giving you advice, so it becomes commonplace. When advice comes from an outside authority, it carries more weight. You want to earn his or her respect. Also, when your parents give you advice it makes you feel like a kid, whereas when an outside authority gives you advice, it makes you feel like an adult."

From then on, whenever the occasion presented itself, I sought out advice for Josh from those I respected. Sometimes, of course, such advice came unsolicited from unexpected quarters, but was useful nonetheless.

One Fourth of July, Leora, Josh, and I went downtown to see the fireworks on the famous D.C. Mall. As we emerged from the subway, Josh ran ahead, and I saw him engaged in conversation with a panhandler, which ended with Josh turning his pockets inside out.

"What was that all about?" I asked when we finally caught up with him.

"The man said to me, 'Give me a dime or I'll punch you in the eye.'

"I told him I didn't have any money on me," Josh said. "He said, 'I don't believe you. Turn your pockets out.'

"So I did. Then he said to me, 'Jeez, boy, don't you know better than to listen to that *sheet*? When someone says that to you, you just keep walking.'"

Advice from a panhandler! As the Talmud says, the wise person is someone who learns something from everyone.

THE NEXT INCIDENT that comes to mind happened when Josh was in high school; his backpack was stolen. The loss of his backpack and a small amount of money was of no great concern. As Elizabeth Bishop says, "Lose something every day." Of far greater concern, his house keys were in the backpack, along with his ID and address—a perfect present for a would-be thief. To make matters worse, Josh had left his backpack in a highly insecure place—hanging from a hook in the hallway.

Although the prospects of getting it back were poor, I felt obliged to go to the school, even though it was after hours, to see whether we could find out anything useful. We were met by the janitor, a large African-American man, sitting in the observation station near the entrance. At a workstation in the office behind him, also within sight of the front door, was a timid-looking woman whom he introduced as his wife.

I told our story, and he offered to look for the backpack and its contents but said we were unlikely to retrieve them. He doubted whether anybody would break into our home, however. The thief was almost certainly another student, who would want only the bag and money.

I must have prompted him to give Josh some advice about how best to take care of his property, which he was happy to do. I certainly did not expect the sermon that followed, though I welcomed it.

"Son," he said, "you have done a careless thing. You have left your possessions in plain sight for anyone who is inclined to pilfer. That is a careless thing to do. And what happened? Sure enough, someone came along and pilfered it. If I was your father, I keeps you *po* for a while.

"Son, trust nobody. I've learned that the hard way. Only her," he said, gesturing to his wife in the back office. "Only *her* do I trust—and not even *her* all the time. And you trust your possessions to a stranger, by leaving them hanging out in plain sight! Son, that's just plain foolish. If I was your father, I keeps you *po* for a while, so that you can learn— money is precious; it's hard to come by.

"One time as a child, I earned some money. I thought I was rich and clever. What happened? I lost it to the flimflam man. I come home to my mother all downcast. She asks me what happened and I tell her I tried to multiply my money with the flimflam man. She gets mad at me and says, 'Son, you acted foolishly. Now to show you the value of money I keeps you *po* for a while.'"

Josh and I left the school with no hope of retrieving the backpack, but enraptured by the janitor's eloquence and passion. Josh had also learned an unforgettable lesson about taking care of his things. As I reflected on the speech, it occurred to me that the janitor's worldview was more mistrustful than my own—but highly useful. I could never have given Josh such a powerful message; nor could the loss have had such a positive effect on him without the janitor's help. And most important, perhaps, Josh had been enriched by hearing a different point of view expressed in a different voice—and so had I.

Although Josh was really a good kid in high school, in his last couple of years he fell in with a wild bunch (at least by my definition). This group was led by a junior whom I will call Al, and it soon became apparent that wherever Al went, trouble followed.

One night Josh didn't come home till daybreak. This was before cell phones, so Leora and I had been up all night worried sick. He told us he had gone downtown with Al and some other kids to a dangerous part of the city. Al parked the car under an overpass, took out a boom box, and proceeded to pass around drugs and dance in the night air. Josh declined the drugs and, feeling uneasy about the situation, told Al he would take the subway home.

Unbeknownst to him, the subway had already stopped running (it must have been past one a.m.), so he decided to wait at a bus stop until the trains began to run. He fell asleep and woke to find his wallet gone. There was another man at the bus stop, who offered Josh a dollar for subway fare home, which he gratefully accepted, even as he tried to suppress the unkind but unavoidable thought that the dollar might have come from his own wallet.

After hours of recovery sleep, Josh woke and we were just discussing the event when the phone rang. It was for Josh: The stranger on the other end of the phone told Josh that the bank had found his bank card. Now all the bank needed to cancel the card, the stranger said, so that nobody could get money from his account was. . . you guessed it, the PIN number. When I got on the phone, it was obvious that the stranger was no bank official, and he quickly hung up.

I called 911 and a huge policeman arrived at our house, bearing a gun and a baton. After he took the history and declared that there was nothing to be done, I asked him whether he would be kind enough to advise Josh as to the wisdom of his behavior the previous night. (The valuable lesson of the school janitor was fresh in my mind.)

"I wouldn't dream of going down to that part of the city late at night," the huge policeman said, "unless I had to do so for work. I'd be terrified. It's bad enough during the day." Josh sat silently, gaping at the policeman, his eyes wide and his pupils dilated. That was another great lesson from a stranger, which might well have saved Josh's life by preventing further forays into danger.

The New Year was approaching and Al invited Josh to an event in Baltimore—"A fantastic happening, you just can't miss it." Leora had by this time delegated to me any decisions that fell under the category of "male adolescent behavior," so Josh came to ask me for permission. The answer was simple: "No."

He was crestfallen. "Why not?" he asked.

I thought of Al with his track record of trouble, culminating in the night under the overpass. Then I cast my mind back farther to my own

reckless adventures: my brush with the South African police, the stab-
bing that nearly killed me, the hepatitis C that came back to haunt me.
How could I condense all this experience for him in a few words? I knew
he would tire quickly of any lecture I might give. Since there was no
scoutmaster or janitor or policeman at hand, which outsider could help
us now? Luckily, I thought of the very person—a poet I had long
respected and enjoyed: W. H. Auden.

"The answer's no," I said to Josh, "because death can come in an
instant. You're heading up the I-95 and it's New Year's Eve, and some
driver's been celebrating too much, and bang! That's it!

"Read W. H. Auden's 'Musée des Beaux Arts,'" I said, "and then let's
discuss it further."

For those of you who are unfamiliar with this poem, it is named
after an art gallery in Brussels that houses a painting depicting the death
of Icarus. You may recall the Greek myth in which an engineer, Daedalus, and his son, Icarus, are held captive on the island of Crete. To escape, Daedalus, the architect of the famous Cretan labyrinth, fashions
wings for himself and his son. The wings are made out of feathers glued
together with beeswax, and Daedalus warns his son not to fly so high
that the sun will melt the wax, nor so low that the ocean spray will soak
the feathers. In either case, the boy would fall into the ocean and
drown. "Take the middle course," the father urges, reflecting the Greek
philosophy of the golden mean, doing things in moderation and avoiding extremes.

Father and son escape as planned, but soon the boy, filled with the
sheer exuberance of flying, ignores his father's advice and flies higher,
higher and higher until the sun melts the wax, and Icarus plummets to
his death in the sea that is now named after him.

Of the painting depicting the death of Icarus, Auden writes:

About suffering they were never wrong,
The Old Masters. . . .

And he proceeds to describe such an ordinary day, with people and animals doing all their ordinary things, paying little heed to

Something amazing, a boy falling out of the sky.

Auden is relaying a profound truth: Tragedy happens even while people are going about their everyday lives. In retrospect, we often say, "We should have seen it coming." At the time, though, everything seemed normal.

To his great credit, Josh read the poem and got the point. He understood my concerns and declined his friend's invitation. Years later, when he was studying college English, Josh was assigned Auden's poem. We read it again together and laughed about the trip to Baltimore that never happened. At that time we had needed advice from an outsider and could not have found a better guide, nor a more eloquent one, than W. H. Auden.

It takes a village to raise a child, or so they say. I have always thought of the expression simply in terms of how much work is involved. But the saying conveys much more than that. Different people offer different points of view, and have different ways of conveying their message. A growing child needs diverse exposures if he or she is to understand and navigate our complex world.

> *Try to learn something from everyone, and (with proper supervision) encourage your children to do the same.*

Chapter 39

Telling a Story

Stories are equipment for living.

—KENNETH BURKE

The two-year-old boy sat in the driver's seat of a fire engine, courtesy of a kindly fireman. The boy worked the steering wheel, honked the horn, and fiddled with anything and everything he could reach. When it was time to leave, as one might expect, he refused. No! No! No! He wanted to stay! His father (Josh) said, "If you come with me and Grandpa, I'll tell you a story about our visit to the fire station." The boy readily relinquished his throne. He then spent the next half hour happily hearing about his morning's adventure, and finally told the story himself. In this simple example, we see how a story enabled a small child to pull himself away from a fascinating machine and transition to the next activity. In addition, the story helped him consolidate the experience and organize another little corner of his mental world.

Stories are so fundamental to human lives that no culture is known that lacks them. Listening to stories, we hang on every word, riveted, and we care about the characters almost as if they were real. Two famous anecdotes—both favorites of mine—bring this intensity home.

When Charles Dickens's *The Old Curiosity Shop* was first published in the United States, it was a serial. Each week's new chapter arrived by ship—and people knew it. When the angelic child heroine, Little Nell, lay at death's door, thousands of New Yorkers met the boat. They simply *had* to know. "Did Little Nell die?" they called up to the ship's crew. "Is Little Nell alive?"

Another famous story is told about a powerful version of *King Lear* produced by the Yiddish Theater in New York City in the early twentieth century. The actor playing Lear, the retired king thrown out of his home by his ungrateful daughters, so moved a woman in the audience that she stood up and chastised the daughters right in the middle of the play. "You should be ashamed of yourselves!" she cried out. Then, turning to Lear, she said, "You can come stay with us if you like."

My topic here, however, is not so much the capacity of stories to divert and move us as on stories as "equipment for living." Most therapists, myself included, believe in the value of creating a personal narrative. This could be a short story, as in how a certain problem (or string of problems) developed. Or it could be a novel that spans one's whole life from childhood to the present day. Time-limited therapies try to wrap things up with a short story, whereas psychoanalysis, with its free associations and open-ended nature, tends to produce longer works, like *Remembrance of Things Past*.

How then does creating a story of one's problems help resolve them? Let's look at one particular type of problem—trauma and its consequences. Severe trauma, such as humiliation, sexual assault, or an enemy's bomb, can lead to severe problems, notably post-traumatic stress disorder (PTSD). People with PTSD may withdraw from friends and family, be overwhelmed with dread and terror, or have trouble sleeping. They may suffer flashbacks or terrible nightmares, and may medicate themselves with drugs or alcohol, which compound their problems.

To make matters worse, many traumatized people have little understanding of how their prior injuries relate to their current problems.
Nothing makes sense, so a better life seems impossible. Among other
things, they need to develop a narrative. They need to construct a story
about how one thing led to another, and another, and another, until
finally here they are with all their suffering—and all their strengths.

Traditionally, such a narrative has evolved as a collaboration between patient and therapist, and therapy remains a useful (sometimes
vital) way to deal with trauma. However, there is an impressive body of
research showing that people can create meaningful and useful narra-
tives on their own. In 1966, James W. Pennebaker, professor and chair
of psychology at the University of Texas in Austin, developed a technique called "the writing exercise," in which people are asked to write
down their deepest thoughts and feelings about something that concerns them. In research on this technique, there are typically four sessions of writing, each about twenty minutes long, spread out over several
days. The subjects are instructed not to bother about grammar or sentence structure—simply to write. The goal is not the written product
but the process of writing itself. Pennebaker's instructions for the
writing exercise, taken from his book *Opening Up*, are reproduced in
the appendix on page 325.

By now there have been hundreds of controlled studies on the writing exercise, yielding many intriguing results. A group of Texas Instruments workers, for example, had undergone a harsh layoff: Their
unexpected job loss was compounded by an impersonal and insulting
process, the kind with security guards escorting them out like thieves.
As you can imagine, the workers were angry.

The company then hired an outplacement firm to help them get
new jobs. A controlled study of the writing exercise was conducted on a
subset of the workers. Those in the control condition were simply asked
to write a report of their day's activities, whereas the experimental
group was to write about their deepest thoughts and feelings. The outcome: Those in the experimental group found new jobs more quickly

than the controls, even though they had made roughly the same number of phone calls and gone to the same number of job interviews.

Pennebaker's theory as to why the study subjects fared better was simple: They weren't as angry, and an angry attitude is a turnoff to prospective employers. The writing times were short and the stories rudimentary, which raised a key question: How could an exercise that seemed so simple have had such a powerful effect? To find out, Pennebaker and his colleagues looked at some of the writing samples. To their surprise, they found that even extremely terse notes could prove helpful. For example, one engineer wrote on the first day, "Thinking about getting new job. Have to tell girlfriend." The next day he wrote, "Writing exercise yesterday was very helpful." How could writing those few simple statements have been helpful? the researchers wondered. It turned out that the man was considering taking a job in another town. He needed to discuss that with his girlfriend, as leaving town would probably end the relationship. Understandably, he had been avoiding that discussion. But the writing exercise—even though he didn't actually write much—forced him to confront his avoidance and tackle the problem head-on. (In the end, he took the job and broke up with his girlfriend.)

Pennebaker then asked whether any specific elements in what people wrote could predict positive changes in their lives. If so, that might explain how the exercise works. The tool here was a computerized linguistic program that analyzes text.

When I ask people to guess what kind of language best predicts life change, they almost always guess words that refer to powerful emotion: words like "rage," "passion," "death," "love," and so on. That would be a reasonable guess, since powerful emotions do get our pulses going. In fact, researchers Larry Cahill and James McGaugh (from the University of California at Irvine) have shown that emotional parts of stories—those parts you would predict would cause the reader or listener to secrete adrenaline—fix those memories in the brain. We remember emotional parts more powerfully than neutral parts of stories. Paradoxically, however, it turns out that when it comes to predicting changes in behavior, cognitive words such as "realized," "understood," or "appreciated for the first time" have the greatest impact.

These findings are consistent with what psychotherapists have observed: People tend to process experiences best, especially traumas, if they are using both the emotional and analytic parts of the brain. It is also a good sign if the story changes over time. We have all encountered people who underwent a trauma and then felt compelled to tell everybody about it again and again. In fact, when I was stabbed in South Africa I felt that sort of compulsion. It was a bit embarrassing to me until I realized that storytelling is a fundamental part of how we deal with trauma. As the story is repeated, however, the perspective should shift if the story is to help a person heal. New details should come into focus; others should recede. Such shifts in language, perception, and perspective all reflect the active mental processing needed to recover from trauma.

Another compelling exercise that uses stories to help people deal with adversity is embedded in a course in mindfulness and self-compassion run by a friend and colleague, Chris Germer, a clinical psychologist affiliated with Harvard Medical School. According to Germer, of all the exercises in the course, one that involves exploring past adversity usually evokes the greatest interest.

In the first part of the exercise, which Germer calls "Silver Linings," the group leader asks participants to reflect on a predicament from their past that seemed insoluble at the time, then its lessons. That's where the silver lining enters the picture: What did they learn from the experience that they could have learned in no other way? In the second part of the exercise, participants tell the story of a current situation that seems insoluble, and share with the group what they've learned from past adversity that might be helpful in their new dilemma.

The first phase of the exercise is intended to guide people to think deeply about their past problems—and how they resolved them—resulting in both insight and a personal sense of competency. The hope is that this newfound feeling of effectiveness will be translated into a sense of optimism and courage as they work through their current situation. According to Germer, "It's as though they discover a resource within themselves that transcends the content of the problem."

What I hope I have shown in this discussion is that whether you are a two-year-old child or a wounded veteran, whether you are suffering from the long-term effects of repeated humiliation or a sudden assault of indescribable violence, language is your friend. When we can label our feelings, we acquire some mastery over them; by understanding the causal connections that have led us to our current fix, we can view the world as a more predictable and less frightening place. All these effects occur when you tell a story, even if nobody else is listening.

The stories you tell both reflect and shape who you are. Therefore, choose your words thoughtfully, but don't be afraid to change your story. Changes often reflect an increasingly subtle and complex understanding of life and its possibilities.

Chapter 40

The Gift of Meditation

Nowhere can a man withdraw to a more untroubled
quietude than in his own soul.

—MARCUS AURELIUS

Meditate. All is full of light, even the night.

—VICTOR HUGO

Although I always try to learn something from every patient, a few
have actually altered the course of my thinking and my career.
One such person was Herb Kern, the scientist I mentioned previously,
whose observations led me and my colleagues to describe seasonal
affective disorder and discover light therapy. Another patient who had
a pivotal influence on my work was a young film student named Paul,
who encouraged me to meditate.

Paul first entered my practice when he was in his mid-twenties, by
which time he had an established diagnosis of severe bipolar disorder,
an illness that had whipsawed him through several gut-wrenching epi-
sodes of mania and depression. I managed to stabilize these mood

swings with a stiff cocktail of medications, but Paul was left feeling emotionally blunted and "not really happy." That was to change when he stumbled upon Transcendental Meditation (TM). Soon he reported to me that he was feeling happy "ninety percent of the time." I told him I had learned the technique decades before but had long since quit. He persuaded me to have my technique refreshed by a seasoned TM teacher, then checked up on me often to make sure I was practicing regularly. It turns out that in order to derive benefit from TM—or, for that matter, from any healthy activity—you have to practice regularly. In short, it has to become a *habit*.

Indeed, once I started to meditate regularly, I noticed many salutary changes. I became less reactive, more patient, and kinder, because I felt less stressed and anxious. These changes were so significant that I soon recommended the technique to several of my patients, with good results. In addition, I undertook research on the technique in two groups: veterans with combat-related post-traumatic stress disorder (PTSD), and people with bipolar disorder. So impressive were the results that most of the clinicians on my team went on to acquire TM training at their own expense. After researching the published literature on TM, I became excited enough to write a book on the subject (*Transcendence*), and, as I mentioned in an earlier chapter, I credit my regular TM practice with giving me the capacity for solitude and sustained creativity that writing a book requires. Recently I asked Paul why he had persisted so in making sure that I returned to TM and practiced regularly. He replied, "I thought that if you did, it would enable you to help many other patients as well." He was right.

According to a Buddhist expression that I love, "There are ten thousand doors to dharma," meaning that there are many ways to virtue. As a psychiatrist, I have known many colleagues who believed that their type of treatment was the best way or even the only way. I raise this caveat here as I do not wish to appear to be following in their footsteps. There are many forms of meditation and other disciplines of the mind that might help people overcome adversity. I am focusing on TM and omitting specific reference to these other techniques because my goal in this book is to report on wisdom drawn from direct personal experience, my own and that of others I have known, not to be encyclopedic or comprehensive.

In *Transcendence*, I told many stories of how TM had helped people to overcome various forms of physical and emotional adversity. Some were severely handicapped by these problems, while others, like myself, were simply grappling with the stresses of a fast-paced life. I came to know three remarkable TMers, however, who formed a category of their own. All three had suffered from the severe triad of drug abuse, imprisonment, and living on the street—a cluster of adversities from which it is nearly impossible to recover. Yet recover they did—and TM, along with other important factors, was central to their feat. I am happy to include their stories here, because they demonstrate that people can recover from unthinkable suffering, and because they show how a subtle technique involving a regular retreat into the self can be a powerful force for change.

A PLAIN SQUAT REDBRICK BUILDING stands somewhere in New York City. Surrounded by a parking lot and a large unpaved yard, with a few benches under some tall trees, the building reminds me of the field clinics I used to visit during my time in the homeland while fulfilling my military service in South Africa so many years ago. Some men sit smoking calmly under the trees, compounding the sense that this establishment has somehow escaped the pulse and drumbeat of this most hectic of cities and fallen into another place and time. The property belongs to a charity founded to help homeless and formerly incarcerated people find their way back into ordinary society.

The center's supervisor, whom I will call Splash, a former resident of the program, has an aura of calm but powerful authority that helps lubricate hundreds of daily interactions among people who have many reasons to feel jumpy. Since he is always looking to acquire new programs for his approximately two hundred men, Splash was delighted when a donor offered Transcendental Meditation to the residents.

When he talks about his work, Splash moves easily between his own story and those of the residents; there are so many convergences. When he first entered the program, he says:

> I had a serious problem with drugs, which caused me to be homeless, incarcerated, and jobless. I was out on the street for about a year. I had burned every bridge possible. Being homeless is a kind of empty feeling. You want to be invisible, but you're not. You hope people don't see you, but deep down inside you know they do. There's always a look they give you—disgust.
>
> Drugs had robbed me of everything, including my self-respect and my dignity. I came in touch with the fact that I'd done this to myself, that there was no one else to blame. I had good parents who gave me a good education and placed me on the right path. And I let the streets and the glitter attract me. And then, when the addiction took over, I was a rat. It was almost like an evil twin came out, and I became who I became.
>
> I was like Dr. Jekyll and Mr. Hyde, and Hyde was pretty bad. No values. The drugs made it okay for me to put aside all the values that I knew. What was wrong, what was right didn't mean anything to me. Age didn't matter. I'm going to use by any means necessary. If you're in the way, you're in the way. That's where the drugs took me. It wasn't always that way, but in the last two years of my life using, there was no more Dr. Jekyll. It was just Mr. Hyde, 24/7. I don't know when he crossed over; it just happened. That was the worst time of my life.

Now, however, that history of drug abuse, homelessness, and incarceration serves to give Splash a special insight into the other residents. He realizes that it's possible to rise up "like the phoenix . . . from an abyss." That journey involves many interventions: a detox program, a twelve-step program, and finally, a way to earn money legally—which is where the program for homeless men entered the picture.

So Splash became clean and sober as a result of his efforts working his twelve-step program. He has his religion, a meaningful job and, finally, a mate and a lovely daughter. What, you might wonder, could TM add to the mix? A great deal, according to Splash.

I hate to say it, but TM is almost like a magic bullet. I say that because the addict is always looking for the magic bullet, which doesn't exist, right? But I would say I felt the effect instantly. I had more energy, more tolerance for my other life [with my family]. This job I have is so demanding that at times when I left here, it was almost like I'd been working on construction all day long. All I wanted to do was to go home, eat something, and not do anything else besides rest and maybe look at the TV.

What TM has done for me is two things: In the morning it gets me going in the right direction. My focus is a little better. But in the evening I get a second wind. TM has given me the energy to go out and play with my daughter and just be more attentive to other people's needs. Now I am able to listen to my mate, and not just for the sake of doing it. And I have a higher tolerance for stuff. Things that used to bug me don't bug me so much. In the past I would start ranting if I saw dishes in the sink. Now I don't get set off so easily. Like the other day, I took my mate to work and she had left her debit card at home. She called me to tell me. Usually I'd rant about that. But I said, "Never mind, it's okay," and I got into the car and went all the way back to get the card and take it to her. And to see the smile on her face when I got there, that was something—and I know that was the direct result of meditation.

"Julian," a short, solidly built man in his early fifties, is one of the men in Splash's program. Although soft-spoken, he has a serious demeanor that automatically elicits respect. He came to the program after three years in the state prison (for assault) and more than eleven years in the federal penitentiary for drug distribution in South Florida. Being in the penitentiary had been so traumatic that he experienced flashbacks while talking to me. His face took on a grim expression and his eyes darted from side to side, as though he were tracking threatening images from those terrible years.

One reason for his landing in the penitentiary (as opposed to the less dire state prison) was Julian's history of multiple assaults. Once there, however, he decided to keep to himself and stay busy working in prison industries, making military articles "for the boys at war in Iraq." He learned to operate many different machines and obtained scholarships for education, "Because I didn't want to make my time in the federal prison stupid time."

When Julian came out of the penitentiary, he was in a deep depression. His psychiatrist put him on the antidepressant Paxil, but it made him anxious and he stopped it. When he learned to meditate, he started to realize that "my depression was neutralizing itself for some reason. The meditation triggers a certain part of the brain and my depression has become mild. I'm able to acknowledge that there's really nothing I can do about certain things that have me depressed," for example, his estrangement from his now adult son. Besides improving his depression, meditation has helped Julian feel better physically. He suffers from a degenerative joint disease, but finds that "TM relieves me of a lot of pain. Maybe it triggers something in my brain that allows me just to not think so much about the pains I'm going through."

Julian says that meditation "has actually relaxed me in all senses of the word." He is convinced that TM has helped him understand the world better and accomplish more. Most important, perhaps, TM has helped Julian break his long-standing tendency to violent impulsiveness. This new patience was sorely tested when he was recently taken to court for sitting in a park that, unbeknownst to him, was off-limits as a precaution against child predators.

When he arrived in court, the judge appeared to be entertaining the crowd. He asked Julian questions that sounded facetious, irrelevant, and insulting: Had Julian ever been charged with the possession of child pornography? Had he been previously accused of sex with a minor? The questioning seemed to go on and on. Formerly, Julian would have been incapable of answering such provocative questions politely. He would have mouthed off and landed up in the county lockup. With the extra reaction time he has enjoyed since learning TM, however, Julian was able to respond calmly to each question. He was sentenced to pay a two-hundred-dollar fine. He later appealed the sentence and the case was dismissed because the policeman involved failed to appear in court. This whole series of events was a huge victory for a man who had previously been unable to turn his back on even the slightest perceived insult or provocation.

Julian is currently studying to become a drug counselor. When he heard what drug counselors earn, he could not believe he could obtain so much money legally. He has begun to smile at people and is surprised when they smile back. Gradually, he is becoming less of a loner. As he puts it, "Everything negative, I believe, through the help of TM, I have been able to turn into something positive." He can't put his finger on how this has happened, "because TM is so easy, such a simple technique."

He never misses an opportunity to meditate, sometimes in unexpected places.

There's times when my lunch break winds up being close to Central Park, and I've gone there and meditated up on the slopes. And I sit down and I listen, I hear the birds in the background, the wind in the trees, you know, while I'm sitting there.

And I meditate. It actually makes me feel great. And it helps me through my day at work. I'm always telling people, "Good afternoon," "Good morning." It feels so good to get feedback from people on the street.

After *Transcendence* was published, I received many letters, but the following letter from a woman named "Helena" is particularly relevant to our present discussion. I called Helena and we spoke at length, but her own words tell her story best:

> *Dear Dr. Rosenthal:*
>
> *I am a new psychologist and an old TM meditator (it will be thirty years in October).*
>
> *I am just finishing your book on TM. I enjoyed it greatly.*
>
> *I am the lucky and blessed protagonist of a TM transformational story as well, and if you would ever need a new testimonial/story of how TM radically transformed a life, I can provide a juicy one.*
>
> *TM has contributed to truly miraculous changes for me.*
>
> *From abuse to addiction to prostitution and violence of all sorts, I experienced a lot in life. These difficult past experiences have put me in a privileged position to help people.*
>
> *TM affords me wisdom, perspective, compassion, peace, patience, brain coherence (very important indeed!), and great meaningfulness, besides so much else.*
>
> *So I thought I'd send a note of appreciation and also joy to see you as part of the TM meditating family . . . !*

To me, the stories of Splash, Julian, and Helena testify not only to the enormous capacity of humans to survive adversity, but also to the fact that we need help to do so. That help includes the kindness and guidance of others, which are often most readily found in programs established to assist the disadvantaged; the opportunity to work and earn money in legal ways—a serious problem for convicts trying to rebuild their lives; and finally, specific tools, such as meditation.

If you are unhappy with your life, consider changing it first from within. Meditation is a powerful tool for self-change, which often leads naturally to positive changes in those around you.

Chapter 41

By Force of Habit

How we spend our days is, of course, how we
spend our lives.

—ANNIE DILLARD

first saw this quote by Annie Dillard on the bulletin board of a church
on Central Park West, and I remember registering a sense of shock at
a connection that—obvious as it should have been—I had not fully appreciated. What we do on a day-to-day basis constitutes the substance of
our lives. It expresses our values and it shapes our goals. The idea is no
doubt ancient wisdom—as we sow, so shall we reap—but like many
things old and wise, it is easily forgotten.

When I was a young man, habits seemed boring to me—the stuff of
middle-aged stodginess. Over the years, my views have shifted. Although I still respect adventure, I have come to regard habits as
absolutely necessary. How else can anyone navigate the complexities of
life? Imagine how impossible life would be if you had to make a decision about every action. "Now, let's see, should I have breakfast today?
And work? Should I go today or not?"

We acquire many habits as children, though we seldom appreciate the process at the time. "Clean your teeth." "Get to bed on time." "Clean up after yourself." Such instructions vary from place to place and home to home, but everywhere they lead to habits that serve us surprisingly well through life. Other habits we are left to form on our own, and that's where things can become tricky.

According to an old joke, there are two kinds of people: those who think you can divide people into two kinds of people, and those who think you can't. A member of the first group would most likely say: "There are two kinds of habits: good ones and bad ones." This typology is simplistic, yet it has a certain validity. To put it simply, good habits enhance your life, while bad habits make it worse. Another difference is that good habits often pay off slowly and over time, yielding cumulative benefits, whereas bad habits usually offer immediate pleasure, often followed by a nasty rebound—like addictions.

Developing Good Habits

Good habits make life easier. For example, I used to be constantly hunting for my keys, until I decided to put them in the same place every time (and taught myself to remember to do it). That done, I now always know where to find my keys. Likewise, I used to forget whether I had locked my car door or not—causing me unnecessary worry—until I developed the habit of locking it every time. While these minor habits are examples of how to make life easier on a daily basis, some healthy habits can make the difference between life and death—like wearing your seat belt, not texting while driving, or holding on to the handrail on a staircase.

How can we help ourselves form habits that serve us, and quit the ones that don't? To understand how habits develop and persist, consider that the brain consists of billions of nerve cells, or neurons, connected to one another at trillions of junctions called synapses. When we develop a habit, we are making a neurological and psychological connection between a cue that triggers a habit (for example, going to the bathroom in the morning), a habitual behavior (brushing our teeth), and its immediate reward (a fresh taste and tingling sensation in the mouth).

Cue, behavior, and reward: Those are the three essentials of any habit. As we enact this sequence, the nerve cells involved in different parts of it fire together, thereby strengthening their connections. As neuroscientists are fond of saying, "Nerves that fire together wire together." In that way, as habits are repeated, the nerves associated with them keep firing together and the wiring gets stronger and stronger. That's why old good habits keep paying off, and also why old bad habits are hard so to break. Whatever we've been doing, we're wired to keep on doing.

That is why one excellent strategy for consolidating a new habit is to link it to a preexisting one—which is already wired. You're simply adding one more set of links. For example, I often counsel patients to take their morning and nighttime medicines at the same time they brush their teeth, which usually works well. It can be more difficult to take medicine in the middle of the day, perhaps because most people have no ingrained noontime habit to serve as an anchor.

There are at least three regions of the brain that are important to the process of forming habits: the regions that regulate pleasure, good judgment, and the actual physical formation of habits. All three are interconnected by neural circuits.

A brain region that is key to regulating pleasure and reward is the nucleus accumbens, which is itself controlled largely by neurons that release the neurotransmitter dopamine. The anti-Parkinsonian drug pramipexole, which boosts dopamine in the brain, sometimes produces an unusual set of side effects—compulsive gambling, eating, shopping, and sexual behavior—providing clear evidence of a link between these particular bad habits (technically diagnosed as impulse control disorder) and altered brain chemistry. When functioning properly and well integrated with the rest of the brain, our pleasure centers drive us to eat nutritious food and make love—actions vital to our survival, individually and as a species. As we all know, however, when pleasure centers run wild, they can cause us and others no end of misery. We see that with addictions, which I'll discuss in more detail below.

The brain region just behind the forehead, known as the prefrontal cortex (PFC) is important for decision making and executive functions. In fact, the PFC has been dubbed the CEO of the brain. In deciding which habits to cultivate and which to break, we rely heavily on our PFC for good judgment. When we try to break bad habits, however, the PFC and the pleasure centers are often locked in battle. You can almost hear the dialogue: "Go for it! Just one more . . ." versus "You've had enough." Resolving such conflicts wisely often means not scolding yourself as to what you *should* do, which is aversive; beating up on yourself— "There I go again"—trains the brain to associate "should do" with guilt and shame, which is emphatically not what you want. Instead, find a way to reward the pleasure centers that don't involve feeding the bad habit—for example, going for a pleasant walk instead of eating another piece of cake.

Finally, deep inside the brain, buried beneath layers of cortex, are primitive structures in a cluster called the basal ganglia. Although these regions are best known for their role in regulating movement (they function abnormally, for example, in people with Parkinson's disease), the basal ganglia are also important in forming habits. Rat studies show that as rats acquire habits (such as navigating mazes), the basal ganglia become more and more active while the rest of the brain is able to rest. Case studies in humans show that in some people who suffer severe memory loss, certain habits—such as the ability to walk around your own familiar block and find your way back home—are retained. That's thanks to the basal ganglia, now acting as an autopilot.

It is the intricate dance, then, among all these various brain centers that helps determine how we spend our days and thus how we spend our lives. One problem with this dance is differences in timing: Certain pleasure responses are rapid, whereas many useful habits take years to pay off. One solution to this dilemma is to add an immediate front-end reward, as manufacturers and advertisers have known for a long time. In his excellent book *The Power of Habit*, author Charles Duhigg uses the example of brushing your teeth, which pays off over the long run by reducing dental decay and gum disease. But a sixty-year promise won't sell much toothpaste. Instead, manufacturers have learned to produce toothpaste that delivers an immediate reward—fresh breath and a tingling oral sensation. It works. And those of us who would like to develop good habits and break bad ones would do well to take note. Find ways to make healthy habits enjoyable and rapidly rewarding, even though their more important payoff will occur only in the long run.

Luckily, the world is full of small pleasures that will do you no harm and may even be helpful. Such pleasures can help you break old habits and form new ones. Gum instead of cigarettes is a classic example of this strategy, but options abound: Call a friend; take the kids to the park; check your e-mail. You choose. Adding rewards to consolidate habits works for industry, and it can work for us too.

Sometimes if you want to develop a new habit, it helps to understand the biology underlying the behaviors involved. For example, I have used knowledge of the biological effects of light and dark to modify my own sleep-wake cycle, allowing me to go to sleep and wake up at regular hours. I make sure I'm exposed to bright light first thing in the morning, and I keep light levels low in the evening. That also means avoiding bright light from computer and TV screens in the hour before bedtime. By using light and dark in this way, it has been easy for me to go to sleep and wake up earlier, which makes me—and many other people—more productive. What causes light to have these effects? The answer lies in the impact of light and dark on the body's rhythms, which are governed by "clocks" inside the brain. For more details about this topic, I refer the interested reader to my book *Winter Blues*.

Sometimes, however, good intentions and knowledge of biology are just not enough. You need something else or, more specifically, *someone* else. When it came to regular exercise (which we all know we need), I was unable to maintain a steady rhythm without the help of my trainer, Stacy, whom I still see after many years and who has become one of my best friends. In fact, the pleasure of her company was the immediate reward that enabled me to persevere over time, thereby reaping the long-term rewards of exercise and her specific expertise.

Once my conditioning had improved, I felt inspired to exercise on my own as well—something I would be unlikely to do without the structure that training provides. In his book, Duhigg urges that we pay attention to "small wins"—the little gains that urge us on to do even better. Training gave me the boost I needed to maintain a steady rhythm of exercise. Likewise, my yoga teacher has spared me many of the aches and pains so common with aging, so I keep doing yoga. I recently enjoyed a big payoff from my investment in training when I was able to scale the majestic ruins at Machu Picchu. As I stood at the top, I feasted on the view of the iconic mountains and contemplated with wonder the huge stone slabs that had been hoisted up the steep slopes with nothing but muscle power, then impeccably aligned. In that moment, I felt grateful not only to the people of this lost civilization but also to my trainer and yoga teacher for enabling me to reach the top and enjoy the view.

A patient once brought me a *New Yorker* cartoon that consisted of two panels. In the first, a drowning man calls to his sheepdog at the edge of the lake, "Lassie, get help!" The next panel shows Lassie lying on an analyst's couch. Jokes aside, there is a lesson here. If you find it difficult to develop a particular good habit on your own, try enlisting help. For me, help with exercise came in the form of a trainer, but a committed exercise buddy, an aerobics class, or a frisky dog that needs to be walked serves many people just as well. Whichever way you choose, finding help may be more practical than trying to rewire your brain circuitry. Paradoxically, by getting help and feeling encouraged to do more on your own, you may end up doing some useful brain rewiring anyway.

The last good habit of mine that I will mention (lest I leave you with the misimpression that I have too many of them) is meditation. As I have described earlier, my twice-daily practice of Transcendental Meditation has helped me become calmer, less reactive, more focused, and more creative than I was five years ago. In addition, the meditation also seems to have programmed a certain rhythm into my nervous system that helps me adhere better to my other healthy habits, and I have heard similar observations from friends and patients. Duhigg refers to habits that have the capacity to promote other habits as *keystone habits*. As he puts it, keystone habits are "habits that start a process that, over time, transforms everything." For me, meditation has had precisely that effect.

Likewise, getting my sleep-wake cycle in order has enabled me to wake up in time to exercise and meditate before starting the workday. Clearly, it has been yet another keystone habit.

Breaking Bad Habits

So much for good habits; let's look at a few bad ones. The other day I went to lunch with a friend, and when it came time for dessert, my companion offered me a bite of her apple-blueberry tart à la mode. I explained to her that a bite would never suffice for me. I would soon be ordering a dessert of my own, and when I got home, I'd raid the kitchen for anything sweet.

My story, a common one, goes back a couple of decades. At that time, the diet in vogue favored low-fat foods, but downplayed the damaging potential of sugar. I tried to avoid fat, but each year I'd pile on a few extra pounds, which added up over time. Every night I would crave frozen yogurt, which, because it was low-fat, seemed allowable. Yet I noticed that I would already be scooping out the second spoonful before I could swallow the first, and I usually wound up with an empty container in hand. Then the next morning at the breakfast table I'd be at it again as the sugary cereal seized control of my pleasure centers, overruled my good judgment, and (reinforced by my habit centers) drove me to mouthful after mouthful.

The results were as unwelcome as they were predictable: My waistline got bigger and bigger. At one point, I even needed suspenders to hold up my trousers. That did it! I started exploring diets that restricted carbohydrate intake, especially the so-called "high-impact" carbs—pure sugar and white starch. On the recommendation of diet doctors, I began to weigh myself each day and write down the weight. At first, I balked at the idea of keeping a record, reasoning (a bit scornfully) that I could certainly remember yesterday's weight. While that was true, I soon realized that writing down my weight each day let me track weight change over time. I could then begin to recognize patterns of what caused me to gain or lose weight, which allowed me to take prompt corrective action.

Now seems like a good moment to put in a plug for writing things down—in general. I no longer regard making notes as a chore. Rather, it gives me permission to forget, since I know I can refer to the written information whenever I need to. Also, the process of writing ensures that I pay more attention to the matter at hand. Finally, writing something down is a sort of commitment. When you add something on your to-do list, it signals a more serious intent than when you say to yourself, "I should get around to doing that sometime." One of my friends succeeded in breaking her addiction to alcohol, thanks largely to keeping a daily journal of her struggles and successes. In my own experience, writing things down is not only a good habit but also a keystone habit: It helps organize and maintain the other good habits in my life.

Under my new low-carb dietary program, I lost significant weight, and have kept those extra pounds off for years. Best of all, it has been easy, because I have not had to depend upon willpower, which research shows soon runs out of steam. As a friend of mine likes to say, "You can get only so far by the white-knuckle method." So I have kept to a good weight not by struggle but by substituting a new set of habits for the bad old ones. In the process, I have also lost the cravings that used to gnaw every night. I never would have believed it could happen, but it did—I have no midnight craving for sweets. Amazing.

My own story reminds me of one of my clients, whom I will call Marie, a woman in her mid-fifties. Marie had lost control of her diet, her weight, and her life because she was routinely overcome by food cravings in the middle of the night. This pattern of eating at night is common, well documented, and difficult to treat. Marie's eating problems reminded me of experiments conducted on birds that were housed in constant lighting conditions and fed at a certain time each day. Although the birds had no clue as to whether it was day or night outside, just before feeding time, they would get excited and start twittering in anticipation. Evidently their body clocks had reset around their one predictable external cue—feeding time.

Had something similar happened to Marie? It occurred to me that one way to view nighttime eating disorder is as a habit, cued by internal processes that were programmed by experience. Might habit explain, I wondered, at least in part, how Marie's problems had developed? If so, what would happen if she could break the habit? Perhaps she would stop craving food in the middle of the night, just as I no longer felt compelled to gorge on frozen yogurt hours after dinner.

Reasoning along these lines, Marie took the opportunity to try an experiment: She planned a ten-day vacation with no easy access to food after dinner. And, indeed, she was able to get over her nighttime cravings and has sustained her new regimen since coming home. When I last met with Marie, she was continuing to lose weight with little effort, was sleeping better, and was more clearheaded during the day, simply because she had succeeded in replacing a bad habit with a good one—regular meals and no midnight feasts.

Another bad habit that used to cause me no end of frustration was procrastination. I would arrive late at airports and have to run to the gate with my carry-ons; or to the theater, jogging on a full stomach to make the opening curtain. As a student, when I had an exam, I would have to pull an all-nighter, something you can get away with only when you're young, and even then at a cost to your nerves—not to mention your grades. Deadlines were also a problem, as I allowed work to stack up so that most of it got squeezed into the last quarter of the time allotted.

Somewhere along the line, the unpleasantness of being late and the anxiety of not getting things done on time must have reached a critical point. I realized how stressful I was making my life for no good reason. In the words of the addiction world, I "hit bottom." So I decided to get to airports early, amble through the bookstore, and enjoy the predictable wait. Likewise, getting to the theater on time nowadays allows me to peruse the program at leisure. What fun! At work, I now routinely divide long-term projects into smaller chunks and create separate deadlines for each chunk. I don't know why it took me so long to figure out these obvious remedies. I was like the grasshopper in Aesop's fable, who played all summer long, heedless of what he would eat when winter came. I had developed the same bad habit: Live now and pay later. Experience has taught me the less stressful habit of paying as I go, which makes life easier and more pleasant.

In thinking about replacing bad habits with good ones—both personally and in my work with clients—the image of a garden often comes to mind. The skilled gardener knows how to get rid of weeds and keep them away by planting flowers or herbs in their place and using mulch.

In the last chapter, you met some people whose lives had been ravaged by addictions, which had landed them on the street and in jail, and had almost cost them their lives. Yet they count themselves as the lucky ones, because they made it back from the hell of addiction into lives that are productive and fulfilling. Many people are not so lucky. Consider the staggering annual death rates in the United States from these different types of addiction: cigarette smoking—443,000; excessive alcohol use—80,000; prescription drug abuse—27,000. One way to think about these addictions is as *really* bad habits. And let's not forget behavioral addictions—to overeating, sex, gambling, and shopping— each of which can create enormous misery. Indeed, for some people, anything that provides a rapid reward has the potential to seize control of the pleasure centers: I have seen addiction become a problem with day trading, computer games, and texting (especially when driving).

It is beyond the scope of our present discussion to go into the many ways to combat addiction, but understanding the force and nature of habits is a good beginning, because it gives us the key: substituting some other reward for the troublesome substance or behavior. Twelve-step programs, modeled after Alcoholics Anonymous, abound, and that is fundamentally how they work. Instead of their addiction, twelve-steppers are encouraged to substitute healthy habits: regular meetings with sober friends and fellows; adhering to a set of principles (the twelve steps) designed to help people stay away from whatever has caused them trouble; and a belief that through an external agent (such as a higher power or the strength of the group), the addiction (bad habit) can be overcome one day at a time.

In less dramatic situations, the same method works—as when I eliminated sugar and Marie broke her nighttime eating habit. But even addictions at this level take time to break. I now enjoy a wide variety of healthy foods that contain very little pure sugar, which once would have seemed like a miserable way to live. It took time to adapt to the new diet, but I actually learned to enjoy it.

Here's the bottom line: Bad habits usually offer quick rewards with a sting in their tail, whereas good habits usually offer gentler rewards that pay off over time. In swapping a bad habit for a good one, you will usually need to wait some time for the old bad habit to lose its grip so you can fully embrace the new one. The belief that things can get better is often what sustains people through this waiting interval.

Developing Good Habits for Organizations

Good habits are important not only for individuals but for organizations as well. My friend Ray Dalio, founder of Bridgewater Associates, currently the largest hedge fund in the world, has outlined the principles that are the intellectual bedrock of the organization (there are about two hundred of them, and they are available online at www.bwater .com/Uploads/FileManager/Principles/Bridgewater-Associates-Ray-Dalio-Principles.pdf).

On reading through these principles, it becomes clear that when they are operationalized, they constitute a set of valuable habits that are clearly key to the success of both the organization and its founder: habits such as radical transparency (most meetings are recorded and available for others to hear) and the pursuit of truth (as opposed to looking good to others). Under a section called "Doing the Tasks," Dalio points out, "I believe the importance of good work habits is vastly underrated," and adds, "It is critical to know each day what you need to do and have the discipline to do it." Consistent with the theme of this book, he emphasizes the need to learn from mistakes and use adversity as a challenge and an opportunity for growth, rather than considering these events as disempowering setbacks.

As for me and bad habits, like most people, I am a work in progress. It is easy to let good habits slip away, and bad habits have a tendency to reassert themselves. I take comfort in the words of Tennyson that "He is all fault who hath no fault at all." Simply understanding, however, the value of good habits in leading a good life is an important step to attaining that life.

> *Good habits can both prevent adversity and help you escape from it. Implementing good habits on a daily basis will help support your long-term goals and sustain your values. If you wish to change bad habits, first seek to understand them as a key to replacing them with good ones. Above all, don't forget to reward yourself, in order to reinforce the new habit.*

Chapter 42

The Quest for Excellence

We are what we repeatedly do. Excellence, then,
is not an act, but a habit.

—ARISTOTLE

Genius is one percent inspiration, ninety-nine
percent perspiration.

—THOMAS EDISON

The first time I ever saw the word "excellent" was as a stamped im-
print on my grade-school report. The principal of our grade school
had two rubber stamps: a square one that said "good work" and a round
one that said "excellent."

My transition from home to elementary school had not been easy—I
screamed when my mother dropped me off on the first day. "Don't worry;
I've got him," said a portly woman teacher, seizing my wrists. I kicked her
as hard as I could, but for all the good it did me, I might as well have
kicked a tree trunk. On the second day, I resisted leaving home so fiercely
that my mother instructed Lucas to pick me up and put me forcibly into

the car. I can still remember the look of sympathetic reluctance in his eyes, but his sympathy did not stop me from biting his forearm—to no avail, of course. For years afterward, Lucas would proudly show me the battle scar he claimed my teeth had left on his skin.

At that point, my parents took me to see the elementary school principal, who was a friend of theirs. He asked me what I enjoyed doing, and his kindly manner was reassuring enough for me to tell the truth. "I like blowing soap bubbles in the bathtub," I said. He smiled and said that was a fine thing to do, but I would not be able to make a living from it when I grew up. Instead, I would need to find some work, just as my father and he had done, and school would help me do that. That made sense. He invited me to check in with him each day en route to class, which he said would make his day happier too. I never took him up on his offer, though. I didn't need to. A little kindness, an explanation, and some reassurance had done the job.

Perhaps because of his kindness, the principal's rubber stamps on my report cards had special weight and meaning to me. I soon learned that "excellent" was better than "good work," so the round stamp was the one I wanted. Years later I learned that one meaning of "excel" is to surpass. I found that interesting because it meant going beyond. Excellence, then, means testing the limits of what you are able to do. I have been fortunate enough to meet in my lifetime many friends, colleagues, and patients who have successfully engaged in a quest for excellence, some of whom you will meet in this chapter.

When we look from afar at people who have accomplished at an extraordinary level, their lives may seem charmed, far indeed from adversity. I would suggest, however, that excellence and adversity are often intimate companions. First, the quest for excellence may be born of adversity. Second, when you pursue excellence, you deliberately make life difficult for yourself—by battling against odds, taking risks, surviving failure, and persevering—as a necessary part of your quest. Finally, when you aim high, adversity will invariably appear, and how you handle it can make all the difference to the outcome.

Let's consider our first case: adversity as a spur to excellence. One of my clients, whom I will call Martin, is a prominent scientist in his mid-sixties, who continues to write prolifically. When I asked him what drives him to excel, he answered without hesitation, "Insecurity from my childhood." Precociously clever in elementary school, Martin was skipped ahead two classes. But then, just as he found his bearings in his new class, he was switched to a more challenging school, where everyone had taken several years of Hebrew, a language that he had never learned before. Add to this mix a father who expected nothing but the best from his children, and you can understand why Martin felt insecure. To overcome these feelings, Martin studied so hard at school that his natural ability took him to the top of the class. "By that time," says Martin, "my work habits had become ingrained, and they have stayed with me for the rest of my life." Martin's story is common, though not all children whose limits are pushed enjoy such a happy outcome.

The quest for excellence invariably involves a conscious choice to accept adversity as part of the cost. "Why do you have to write another book?" Leora used to ask me. "Or take on all these other tasks? Why do you have to make life difficult for yourself?" I had no answer at that time, but now we both understand that it is just part of my nature to pursue goals beyond my reach. Whenever I do reach my goal, I seem to move the goalposts a little farther away. The psychologist Abraham Maslow describes such behavior as coming from a privileged but basic human need to "self-actualize," to achieve a full expression of one's skills or talents. As Maslow put it, "Musicians must make music, artists must paint, poets must write if they are to be ultimately at peace with themselves." Such people, however, demand much of themselves and struggle compulsively to get things "just right"—which invariably involves adversity, as things often go wrong (that's a given in life) or fall short of expectations. The work then has to be reconceptualized, revised, or redone.

My friend and trainer Stacy King is an example of someone constantly in pursuit of excellence. Not only is she superb at her profession but she continually strives to sharpen her core techniques and learn new ones. In interviewing her, I was not surprised to learn that she has consciously pursued excellence since her early years. As a child, Stacy was on track to become a professional athlete, a form of excellence with its own special flavor, because both the sacrifices and the glories are right out in front, highly visible. So let's look at the trade-offs from this point of view.

Stacy became a competitive gymnast at age eight, after which, for the next fifteen years, she trained for many hours each day. In the process she missed much of the ordinary fun that schoolgirls enjoy, such as hanging out with friends or watching TV (the Internet was not yet invented). Yet she maintained her pursuit, undaunted by broken joints (and surgeries), herniated disks, and ongoing pain. When it became clear that although a superb gymnast, Stacy was not going to make it to the Olympics, she shifted her goals and used her gymnastics to obtain a full scholarship to a level-one university. Now a physiotherapist, she often works with gymnasts. She helps them to realize their dreams, but also to adjust to reality if it turns out that they are not among the lucky few who make it to the highest tier.

Stacy's story will be familiar to many competitive athletes. Attaining excellence in *any* field requires devoting thousands of hours to perfecting the craft, and athletics is no exception. In the process, athletes forgo many of life's simple pleasures. Injuries are common, and success at the highest levels is rare. When they are children and adolescents, their sacrifices are matched by those of their families, who spend hundreds of hours shuttling children to and from lessons, meets, games, and other sports-related events. The financial costs are also substantial. It's true that these costs are offset by the huge sums earned by those few sports stars who reach the apex, but players of the year and Olympic medalists are rare birds indeed.

Even when athletes do reach the top, it is a continual challenge to stay there. The years of sacrifice can weigh heavily, as do fears of losing their edge (which is inevitable as the years progress). How they deal with these challenges—which are often psychological—makes all the difference to the outcome. When Trevor Immelman, the South African golfer, was competing against Tiger Woods to win the 2008 Masters, he received a voice-mail message from his golf hero, the legendary Gary Player, that gave him goose bumps. According to Immelman, "Mr. Player told me he believed in me and I needed to believe in myself. He told me to just go out there and be strong through adversity, because he said that adversity would come and I would just have to deal with it. I took that to heart, and I'm obviously thankful for the message." Immelman went on to beat Woods and win the Masters.

The message that Player gave Immelman is profoundly important not only for the game of golf but for the game of life. Ray Dalio, founder of the world's biggest hedge fund, echoes Player's message: "Successful people," he says, "understand that bad things come at everyone and it is their responsibility to make their lives what they want them to be by successfully dealing with whatever challenges they face." I have heard the almost identical message, with minor variations in wording, from people at the top in many fields of endeavor.

It is also invaluable in many fields, sports included, to have a mentor—someone who can help you get to the top and stay there. Although obstacles to success can be technical in nature, often they are psychological, and it was the psychological challenge—specifically anticipating adversity and handling it when it arises—that was the focus of Player's advice to Immelman.

There is a fine line, however, between believing in yourself, which is conducive to excellence, and thinking too well of yourself, which is not. A friend of mine, Barry Zito, an award-winning major-league pitcher, recognizes that when he begins to "dig myself too much," he is allowing his ego to interfere with his quest for excellence. This problem can occur in many different fields of endeavor. In the movies, for example, I have noticed that many talented Hollywood actors fall short of real excellence because they appear to dig themselves too much and are therefore unable to lose themselves in their roles.

Likewise, professionals of all types will attain excellence only if they are able to dig their clients more than themselves. My friend Hilda Ochoa-Brillembourg, founder and CEO of a highly successful portfolio-management group, offers advice that is in line with these conclusions: "Don't focus on the self," she advises, "but on the goal." She adds, "The more you focus on the client, the more you will promote behaviors that will result in excellence."

In all these different areas and more, the quest for excellence requires subordinating the ego to the process or the product. The higher the level of performance required, the more preoccupation with yourself becomes a distraction and a barrier to excellence.

I asked Hilda whether she has been discriminated against as a woman and a foreigner (she was born in Venezuela), to which she responded: "Everybody gets discriminated against. I don't take it personally, lick my wounds, and see myself as a victim—even if I have, in fact, been victimized. And if people discriminate against you, who knows why they are doing that? Of course I feel pain when it happens—anybody would—but I get over it and don't carry grudges. I hope and expect that my competitive advantage will prevail most of the time, but ultimately you have to live with yourself. So your own behavior matters as much to yourself as to your external success." This sort of mind-set is conducive to excellence.

When I asked my friend the artist and filmmaker David Lynch what he thought about the gift of adversity, he said it reminded him of two things: sawing wood and making movies.

I like sawing wood, especially pine, because of the smell it makes when you cut it. There is something beautiful about the saw being pushed through the wood: the sound, the smell, the rhythm. Although the teeth of the saw are sharp, the resistance of the wood is like adversity. The experience wouldn't be the same if it were easy, like a knife going through butter. There's something thrilling about overcoming resistance, overcoming adversity.

Lynch describes the challenge of making a movie, with all the elements that involves:

> The film itself involves lots of other people and lots of money. Big money brings pressure, as do lots of people. You need to get everyone on the same track. In the beginning it feels like you're facing a giant gorge. You start building a glass bridge across that gorge—which is just waiting below with all its rocks and rapids—and you know that the bridge could come crashing down at any moment. At day's end, however, if you get what you're looking for, the glass bridge turns to steel—until the next day, when you start building the glass bridge all over again.

For Lynch as an artist of film, it is vitally important to get "final cut," which means final say as to all elements of the movie that the public ends up seeing. Nowadays, it is difficult for a director to get final cut, because those who have invested huge sums of money in the movie want to be sure that it has, in their opinion, maximum commercial potential. Lynch has learned the hard way, however, not to give in on this point. He explains:

> When I made the film *Dune*, I knew when I signed the contract that I wasn't getting final cut. A lot of me said, "Don't do it," yet I signed on. The movie took three years to make and I died twice at the end because it wasn't the movie I wanted *and* it didn't go down well with audiences. Although I knew beforehand not to sign on to a movie where I didn't get final cut, it took that final adversity to drive the lesson home.

Movie producer Colin Vaines observes that excellence in making movies often requires taking risks. "You can't push the envelope without experimentation. To create an excellent movie you need to reach for something fresh rather than settling for blandness because it's worked in the past." Repeating yourself and settling for a comfortable formula is the biggest recipe for failure. Vaines points out, "Stanley Kubrick pushed the envelope when he made *The Shining*. At the time, Jack Nicholson's performance was criticized as being over-the-top. Kubrick had pushed both Nicholson and himself, going sixty takes when necessary, to elicit that extremely intense performance—which is one reason the film has stood the test of time."

Writers, too, routinely go through multiple efforts before they are satisfied. Ernest Hemingway perhaps put it most succinctly when he said, "All first drafts are shit." I find these words, coming from a master, comforting. I also enjoyed reading Christopher Isherwood's observation that his first draft was generally so bad that it would shock him into writing a better second draft. To his credit, Isherwood took advantage of adversity, using his disgust at the first draft to propel himself forward.

All prospective authors would do well to heed the advice of these masters: Don't worry about your first efforts. Many people are afraid to commit themselves to the written word; they write but never send out their work because they fear being judged and found wanting. That is because they confuse their words with themselves, so that being edited strikes them as a blow to the ego, not a helping hand. A person who can't get past that may never write anything at all, which is a shame: Their unique message to the world will never be delivered.

Elise Hancock, formerly editor in chief of *Johns Hopkins Magazine* and author of *Ideas into Words,* has this advice for those who suffer from a fear of writing: "Remember the many times you've tackled something new. Think hard about how you struggled at the beginning—when you first learned to drive, to kick a soccer ball, or to read a book. In just the same way, when it comes to writing, you're learning—so give yourself a learner's permit. As with many things we fear, it gets easier as you go along. The process may seem like a mess, but all that matters in the end is the finished product." I have taken comfort from similar advice given by the great writer Isak Dinesen, who wrote, "When you have a great and difficult task, something perhaps almost impossible, if you only work a little at a time, every day a little, suddenly the work will finish itself."

A patient of mine, Sam, a highly successful entrepreneur, believes that someone who has gone through adversity—even outright failure—is probably better off than someone who hasn't, as long as the person has learned from the experience. In Sam's opinion, "Such a person is more likely to be empathic, better able to take a broader view of what's happening before reacting." As a manager, all else being equal, Sam will routinely hire a survivor over someone who has never experienced significant trouble. The United States is, Sam says, "the land of the second chances." He cites Steve Jobs as an excellent example of someone who was fired and came back "with both guns blazing." He says there are "loads of such people in the venture capital world."

In pursuing excellence, then, you need to be willing to take calculated risks—including the risk of failure. Also, you need to make the most of failure—to squeeze the lessons out of it, and persevere.

Thomas Edison is quoted as saying, "If I find ten thousand ways something won't work, I haven't failed. I am not discouraged, because every wrong attempt discarded is another step forward."

Sam grew up in a poor family and believes that actually gave him certain advantages. "Poor people tend to speak their mind," he says, "which teaches you how people think. In upper-middle-class settings, on the other hand, people are much more mindful of what they say. They weigh their words carefully." Sam has experienced several serious depressions, which are now fortunately under control. He believes these struggles, too, have given him strength, and he is proud that he has been able to function despite his illness.

Sam points out that he could have made much more money than he did, but that money was not his sole objective. Instead, he has spent years in public service and as a philanthropist. This service aspect of his life has been deeply fulfilling, which illustrates that excellence, like so many things, is a subjective quality. In pursuing excellence, we have to decide what it is that *we* value, not just what others value.

LET ME CONCLUDE by reminding you of one of my favorite quotes, by Aristotle, shown at the chapter head. "We are what we repeatedly do," he said. "Excellence, then, is not an act, but a habit."

Aristotle's insightful words remind me of the Academy Award acceptance speech given by the great actress Helen Mirren for her performance in *The Queen*, in which she portrayed Elizabeth II. In her speech, she toasted the queen as follows:

> Now, you know for fifty years and more Elizabeth Windsor has maintained her dignity, her sense of duty, and her hairstyle. She's had her feet firmly planted on the ground, her hat on her head, her handbag on her arm, and she's weathered many, many storms. And I salute her courage and her consistency.

Like the actress herself, the queen has clearly mastered her art and, day after day, turns in a stellar performance—an example of excellence if ever there was one!

Whatever you choose to do in life, do it as well as you can. There is great joy to be had in the quest for excellence. But be prepared for the adversity that is bound to arise along the way, and remember that how you deal with that adversity will make all the difference to the outcome.

PART III

HEROES

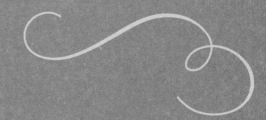

Chapter 43

Death in the Desert

Show me a hero and I'll write you a tragedy.

—F. SCOTT FITZGERALD

Heroes have always intrigued me, perhaps because I was named after one—my uncle Norman, who is the chief subject of this chapter and to whom this book is dedicated.

Everyone, it seems, is fascinated by world-size heroes, such as Winston Churchill and Nelson Mandela, but aside from such massively heroic figures, many of us are proud to have been associated with heroes on a smaller scale. I know I am.

I have chosen for this section four people with whom I've had some personal connection. All were extremely brave; all have my admiration. Some, like my mother or my cousin, I knew well. One, Viktor Frankl, I met only once, but what a meeting it was! And one I never met at all— my uncle Norman.

Frankl, of course, is justifiably a hero to millions. (We will meet him later in this section.) I have included my other heroes alongside him, not only because they're family but because they represent the millions of people who carry out unsung acts of heroism every day. You may well have heroes in your own family—people who faced extreme adversity with courage, generosity, and presence of mind. That is the spirit and the human capacity that this book seeks to understand and celebrate.

IN EARLIER CHAPTERS, I have told you that my uncle Norman was an outstanding sportsman, but really, he was far more than that. His photograph hung prominently in my father's office for all the years I can remember: a handsome man, forever young, with clean features and a mustache. He is sporting the feathered beret of the First South African Irish, the regiment he joined in World War II.

Norman's life was short. He died before his twenty-second birthday.

Although from time to time I would ask my father about Norman, I never did succeed in getting a rounded picture of the man. Most of what little I know comes to me from my cousin Rusty, who was ten years old when Norman died and remembers him very fondly. Norman was an unassuming, friendly man, he says—good-natured enough to take his kid cousin along with him to rugby matches, and perhaps too modest about his own prowess.

I know that at least one woman loved him, and that one comrade and friend held him very dear and never forgot him. Once a year, on Armistice Day, the friend would arrive at our house and pick up my father; the two would go to the cemetery together, where a memorial service was held for those slain in the war. Afterward the friend might stop by briefly for a cup of tea, but these were not occasions for a visit. Rather, they were ceremonies of grim remembrance, unleavened by joy or laughter. This close friend's daughter recently reached out to me on Facebook, where she reminded me of the connection: She also had been named after her father's slain friend; her middle name is Norma.

My late aunt told me that my uncle Norman was not as smart as his older brothers, one of whom became a doctor and the other (my father) a lawyer. They were commissioned officers during the war, which kept them from the firing line. Uncle Norman, however, had elected not to go to college. He went to work in his uncle's polish manufacturing company, where he was a production manager. When war broke out, he joined the infantry.

With his regiment, he was sent to North Africa to support the Allies in their fight against the German forces, led by Field Marshal Rommel, "the Desert Fox." There must have been some downtime in Libya, as Norman played rugby there, South Africans against New Zealanders. But whatever respite the soldiers had was short-lived. A series of fierce tank battles ensued, both sides vying to control North Africa, a major gateway to occupied Europe.

Norman sent Rusty's mother a banner of the First South African Irish regiment in which he served. In silver thread against a black velvet background he had embroidered a harp, a crown, and a shamrock, and the words, "With Love from Norman." In the four corners of the banner are the names of the four battles in which he had already fought: El Gumu, Hobok, Mega, and Banno.

But Norman's luck ran out at Sidi Rezegh in Libya, where a tank battle occurred in which he was fatally injured. We have a better record of his death than his life, thanks to a field chaplain who witnessed it and related the story to a South African reporter, Colin Legum. Legum's article, published in a 1943 edition of the journal *Forward* (long since discontinued) was called "Politics and Rugby."

To give you a context for the article: the Diggers Rugby Club (mentioned below) had become a pro-Nazi organization, and after Norman left the club, no Jew ever played for them again. Many rugby players were Afrikaners, who bore an ancestral hatred for the British. They saw the fight against Nazi Germany as a British cause, and many therefore supported the Nazis. Given this history, it is not surprising that the head of the Diggers Rugby Club did not wish to contribute any money collected from spectators at the stadium gates to the war cause. Mistrust between British and Afrikaans South Africans was bilateral. In fact, so little trust did South Africa's British rulers have in Afrikaner leaders that they actually interned some of them in prisoner-of-war camps, including the future prime minister, Balthazar Johannes Vorster. They feared the Afrikaners would provide intelligence to the enemy.

Here, then, is Colin Legum's piece:

Politics and Rugby: And an Epic of the War

The Diggers Rugby Club held its annual meeting this week. Under the leadership of forward J. Klopper, there was a great deal of talk about politics and rugby, as a result of which the Club declared itself against War Funds benefiting from rugby "gates."

According to the "Daily Mail" report, Mr. Klopper said that "he was not concerned with the war; it could go on for ever so far as he was concerned."

This was a very generous concession on his part.

No mention was made, when the motions of condolences were passed, of the Diggers' Club members who had lost their lives on active service.

This, I presume, is one way of keeping "politics out of rugby."

In the 1941 season Klopper had as a team-mate a promising young full-back who had just turned twenty. Norman Rosenthal was playing his first season of big rugby.

It was also his last season.

The war was some concern of Norman's. He joined the Irish Regiment and saw service in Abyssinia and Libya. His was one of the regiments which found itself surrounded by the Afrika Korps on the bleak desert plains of Sidi Rezegh.

All day long the Luftwaffe swept down and pounded the trapped South Africans: heavy artillery pounded the Springboks furiously and without pause; then the notorious Panzer divisions broke through.

Norman, a sergeant, was in charge of a small company of men sheltering in a slit trench. When the fighting was at its worst he lifted himself out of the safety of the trench to see what chance of escape there was for his men.

He fell back mortally wounded; a bullet-wound in his head and a bullet in his stomach.

Later his men carried him to the emergency field hospital. He was still conscious. The doctors took one hasty look at him and advised the field padre that there was no hope.

The padre takes the story up at this point.

Through a hectic day of fighting Norman had had only a small ration of water; for hours he had been bleeding to death in the pitiless desert heat. The Springboks' water supplies were very low and only small quantities were available for the wounded.

A little of this water was brought to Norman where he lay dying on the battlefield of Sidi Rezegh.

He smiled weakly and told the padre: "It can't do me any good; give it to someone who has a chance of living . . ."

And no amount of persuasion would make him change his mind; he refused the water that could have alleviated his mortal pain.

He had one further request to make to the padre:

"In my pocket you'll find a few pounds; please distribute it among my comrades."

Norman Rosenthal did not die that night; unconsciousness set in and for three days he wrestled with death.

He lies buried beneath a wooden cross somewhere on the tragic battlefield of Sidi Rezegh . . . a young Springbok of twenty-one.

Of him the padre says: "He set an example which is un-equalled in my experience of war; he was the most courageous man I ever saw."

So far as J. Klopper is concerned the war can go on forever.

And so far as the Diggers' Club is concerned, Norman Rosenthal, their promising young full-back, may never have existed.

- The Press devoted twelve inches of space to a report on the views of the champion of rugby—J. Klopper.

- It devoted one line—in the Honours Roll—to Norman Rosenthal, who died that the rugby fields of South Africa might remain safe for the youth of South Africa, Klopper included.—Colin Legum

Norman's remains lie in the Knightsbridge War Cemetery in Acroma, Libya. The makeshift grave marker has been replaced by a granite headstone that records his name in Hebrew, along with the names of his parents and the dates of his birth and death. It notes, too, that he died a hero's death. In all directions, thousands of similar tombstones sweep out across the desert sands, representing the slain troops of many nations and religions. After the war there had been some discussion of repatriating these remains to the soldiers' various home countries, but their families felt that those who had fought together should remain buried together.

Here, then, is my first hero, a man whose life was short but whose death was noble. Had it not been for a field padre and an astute reporter, the story of his courage and his generosity of spirit would have been lost in the desert sands. Even now, eighty years after the event, seeing the story on the printed page never ceases to move me to tears. Such was the nature of the man and his fate. Such is the power of the written word.

> *How long you live is not the only thing that matters; it's also how you live, and how you die.*

Chapter 44

High-Stakes Negotiations at Midnight

Just to be is a blessing. Just to live is holy.

—ABRAHAM JOSHUA HESCHEL

In the years after I left Johannesburg, it became an increasingly violent city, and remains so today. I once tallied up the assaults that my mother had sustained to her person and property, and came up with the number five. In roughly increasing order of violence and violation, they included having her purse snatched at a restaurant; watching her car being stolen out from under her nose as she stood at her kitchen window; having a gold chain snatched off her neck while she was walking in the street; being carjacked at gunpoint; and the incident that I am about to recount.

After my father died, Mom and my sister, Jenny, who remained in South Africa, concluded that it was too dangerous for her to stay on alone in the family home. So they built a spacious cottage for her in my sister's garden. The cottage had a large living room in which Mom conducted bridge classes (she was a champion at the game), and from which she had a wide-angle view of my sister's rich and varied African garden. Many birds fed there, notably the hadeda ibis and the gray go-away birds, named for their respective calls: "Ha-dee-da!" and "Go away!"

The issue of security came up early in planning. Burglar bars for the cottage were, of course, mandatory, plus a panic button. When pressed, it would set off an alarm in the main house. Also, my sister's garden was surrounded by a tall wall, with razor wire on top. That seemed like enough.

Of course, it wasn't. One night, after eating dinner at Jenny's house, Mom returned home to her cottage. She was in her mid-seventies at the time. All was quiet. She made ready for bed and fell into a deep sleep, till she was awakened in the middle of the night to find three young men on top of her—attacking her, squeezing her, choking her, wrenching her rings off her fingers. Despite having her windpipe almost completely choked, she managed to whisper, "If you get off me, I will show you where the money is. Then you can leave. Nobody will see you."

It is almost unimaginable that three young men in the dark, having broken and entered, and attacked an old lady, would suddenly stop and listen to her. But they did. They climbed off her. She wandered over to where a large wad of money was hidden and gave it to them.

"Now, I am not turning on the light," she said. "Nobody has seen your faces. That's where the door is. Take the money and go."

And they did.

It took Mom a while to realize that she was actually alone. After the door closed, she steadied herself against the closet while a great wave of sadness passed over her. "I'll never see my children again," she thought. But then all was silent, and she realized that the men in fact had left. She staggered over to the panic button and pushed it long and hard.

JENNY AND HER FAMILY came running over, called a doctor and the police, and took Mom to the main house. As she made her way across a patch of lawn, Mom saw that one of the assailants had left his tattered old sneakers outside her front door. He had stolen her Reeboks! The ones she loved to walk around in! Somehow, in the midst of all the horror—the violation of her space and person, the theft, the threat to her life—that detail registered out of all proportion to its importance. That's what really made her furious—they had stolen her Reeboks! That was the final insult.

The police came quickly. My mother, of course, had no useful identifying information. They examined her cottage and found that the burglar bars had been sawn through. The invaders must have done that while Mom was eating dinner at Jenny's, lain in wait till she slept, then launched their attack. The police seemed unsurprised. "There is nothing unusual about the crime," they said, "except for one thing: The victim is alive."

The doctor came and gave Mom a sedative, and she slipped into a long, chemically induced sleep.

The next day there was a tennis tournament in Johannesburg. Mom loved tennis and the family had tickets. Since she was badly bruised, however, on both her face and body, and had suffered an overwhelming trauma, the family suggested that maybe she'd rather stay home. Mom demurred. She would not let thugs interfere with her enjoyments, she insisted. She would not allow them to control her life. And if others saw how badly she had been injured, well, that was the reality of life in Johannesburg. So off they went to watch tennis.

Mom recovered gradually, both physically and emotionally. She slept in the main house for a while. An electric fence was added to the wall and the razor wire. An armed guard was hired to watch over a small cluster of homes. A tree close to the outer fence was cut down. One by one, the gaps in the system were plugged and Mom moved back to her cottage.

Sometime later, on a visit to Johannesburg, I wondered about a necklace that I had bought her on behalf of my sisters and myself for her seventieth birthday. She'd been so delighted with it! "What happened to the necklace from Rio?" I asked her. "Did the thugs get that as well?"

"Don't be silly," she replied. "The necklace was somewhere else. I had no intention of giving it to them."

And that was the last word on the matter from a champion bridge player and a champion negotiator.

> *Bad things happen all the time, but even if you are in fact a victim, try not to define yourself as such. Retain as much power over yourself as you can, and cede as little as possible to those who would harm you.*

Chapter 45

A Cousin in Trouble

It was a time when a gesture could cost you your life.

—HEINRICH BÖLL, *BILLIARDS AT HALF-PAST NINE*

When the security police pulled a twenty-one-year-old undergraduate out of class at the University of the Witwatersrand in Johannesburg, and arrested him under Section 6 of the Terrorism Act, the young man was stunned. He could not believe he'd been detained. Why? Why would they? He had socialized with black writers, journalists, and poets, some of whom had already been arrested, but so what? He had done nothing wrong, nothing whatsoever, except own a few forbidden books. Well, he had provided a bed overnight to an occasional black activist. But this was his own country, after all, in which he had lived and felt at home most of his life, and he had done no wrong to anyone. He was dumbfounded.

The arrested man was my cousin and childhood friend John Schlapobersky. It was June 1969—Friday the thirteenth, to be exact—and John had no idea what was about to happen. It had never occurred to him that he might be at risk.

He was taken to the headquarters of the security police in Pretoria, the notorious Compol Building, where they locked him in a tiny room and interrogated him continuously for nearly a week, depriving him of sleep for most of that time. Here he met one of the archcriminals of the apartheid regime, Major Theunis Swanepoel, whom he describes as "a nightmarish man—short, stocky, and full of apoplectic fury—who, together with others, smashed and beat me, pulled my hair and beard, and overwhelmed me."

John kept his head, nonetheless: The first phase of his torture, this overwhelming group attack, took place in Afrikaans, the interrogators' language, which John knew and understood. Instinctively, however, he replied in English. He said, "If you want me to answer your questions, you'll have to speak to me in English, as I don't understand a word you're saying." This enraged them further, and he was beaten some more. From then on, though, they spoke to him in English, and they would later discuss him and their strategies in front of him in Afrikaans, not realizing he understood every word. These events were his first small victory, one he experienced as salvation. Now he knew he *could* resist. He knew because he'd done it.

In the second phase of his torture they interrogated him around the clock, working in teams of two. Each team questioned him in a four-hour shift, to be then relieved by another. For John, though, from the Friday on which they began until Wednesday of the following week, there was little relief. During these six days and five nights he had virtually no sleep. For the first four days they had him stand on a brick and allowed him to sit down only for meals and to go to the toilet.

JOHN WAS SUFFERING the particular fate of a naïf aged twenty-one, caught in a political cross fire between government and activists. In the account he recently gave me, drawing on his later experience as a clinician working with survivors, he told me how carefully activists are trained to deal with torturers and interrogators. Trained, they know how to derive strength from their mission; they can feel vindicated and even emboldened by their experiences in prison.

John, however, was not part of an underground movement, had no special training, and was openly contemptuous of his interrogators—which only provoked them. In all, his reactions were so unusual that the security police were convinced they must have caught a very, *very* clever operative, someone connected with high-level black activists and Communists.

As John points out: "The most vulnerable people in a political conflict are those on the margins, because they don't have the ideology to support them in this trauma."

What many people don't appreciate is that sleep deprivation is, all by itself, a form of torture. Consider what the former Israeli prime minister Menachem Begin wrote about his torture at the hands of the Soviets in his book *White Nights: The Story of a Prisoner in Russia.*

> In the head of the interrogated prisoner, a haze begins to form. His spirit is wearied to death, his legs are unsteady, and he has one sole desire: to sleep. . . . Anyone who has experienced this desire knows that not even hunger and thirst are comparable with it.
>
> I came across prisoners who signed what they were ordered to sign, only to get what the interrogator promised them.
>
> He did not promise them their liberty; he did not promise them food to sate themselves. He promised them—if they signed—uninterrupted sleep! And, having signed, there was nothing in the world that could move them to risk again such nights and such days.

John, who has since trained as a psychotherapist and is now a leading clinician in the field of trauma, provides a clinical slant on the effects of sleep deprivation, drawing on his own experience:

I was kept without sleep for about a week in all. I can remember the details of the experience, although it took place forty-three years ago. After two nights without sleep the hallucinations start, and after three nights people are having dreams while fairly awake, which is a form of psychosis.

By the week's end, people lose their orientation in place and time—the people you're speaking to become people from your past; a window might become a view of the sea seen in your younger days. To deprive someone of sleep is to tamper with their equilibrium and their sanity.

In the third phase, the team allowed John to sleep for a few hours. Then in the final, fourth phase, they resumed interrogation for another two days, during which he was allowed to sit.

At this point you may be wondering: If John was innocent and knew nothing, how did the security police come to arrest him in the first place? Why were they going to all this trouble to extract information if indeed he had none? These were the kinds of questions that many South African whites might well have asked at the time, as they went about their comfortable lives. There were probably some who said, "He must have done something to deserve it."

Yet all the evidence indicates that official miscarriage of justice— such as what happened to John—was widespread. Best estimates now indicate that between 1960 and 1989, some seventy-three thousand South Africans were imprisoned without trial. At least sixty-eight people died in detention. How could so many of us have been in such denial? I ask to this day. But then I wonder, What could we have done had we known? Besides, in a way, we *must* have known, because everyone was terrified. Life for us in South Africa was much as Heinrich Böll described life for ordinary Germans during the Nazi era: "It was a time when a gesture could cost you your life."

And John had made many such gestures. He made friends across the color bar, and he opened his home to fellow writers from the townships—

and it almost cost him his life. When these friends were imprisoned, tortured in even more brutal ways, and asked to name names, they named John. You can hardly blame them.

John is convinced that it was thanks only to his immediate family and the lawyers they instructed (to whom he had no access) that the security machine eased up. John had been raised in Swaziland, then a British protectorate, and carried a British passport. So the British ambassador came forward, and pressure was also applied by the South African Jewish community and the Israeli government. All this pressure did not immediately set him free, but John believes it explains why the security police did not advance to their usual next means of torture—electricity—and why he was eventually released.

Instead, after interrogating him for the week, they put him in solitary confinement in the high-security prison called "the Hanging Jail." John spent nearly two months alone in a cell above the condemned men. In the evenings he would hear those awaiting execution singing through the night. On the mornings following the dawn hangings, there would be a dreadful silence in his part of the prison. John had half an hour per day for exercise in a yard that still bore the bullet holes from executions carried out against the wall during the First World War; he had half an hour for showering.

What helped the most, he says, was writing down his thoughts and feelings. He kept a diary on some toilet paper with a pen he had stolen from the interrogation room. Another source of comfort was the Bible. When his home was ransacked at his arrest, the police confiscated many of his books, but allowed him to take his old school Bible into detention. John read it through carefully three times during his detention, and he used its flyleaves and inside covers to create another diary in code about his experience in prison. This Bible is now on permanent display in London's Jewish Museum.

A critical phase of the ordeal began when his jailers found his toilet-paper diary. His own interpretation of their conduct, later confirmed by his family's lawyers, was that the police had come to see they'd made a mistake, yet they couldn't release him—he'd seen too much. And now he was writing it down!

They started leaving a razor blade out for him when he went to shower—a daily invitation to kill himself. Or perhaps there might be an "accident"—like the "accident" that one African detainee had recently suffered in that wing. He had died of a head injury sustained—so the prison doctor said—after slipping on a piece of soap in the bathroom.

Throughout, John fought back in whatever ways he could, beginning when he got them to talk to him in English. Now he persisted in his daily writing, even though he went to bed each night half expecting to be murdered in the dark. Lying awake, his body tensing at every sound, he drew comfort from the heroism of our great-uncle Tzadik, who had taken some of his captors with him to the grave in the killing fields of Lithuania.

After one week in solitary, John was allowed a visit by his parents, who were told to bring him a change of clothing. Until then, he'd had no idea of the efforts they were making—first to visit him, then to secure his release. The "privilege" of a visit was the first sign of hope, but it was nearly two months before he saw them again. During those two months he believed the security police were weighing the option of his execution.

Eventually, John was given a choice: Stay in prison and continue his studies by correspondence (while those he was arrested with were put on trial), or take a plane to Israel. It was a no-brainer, really. But first he had to face another figure in South Africa's panoply of grim characters. Before he left, the infamous Major (and later General) Johan Coetzee spent days going through his interrogation records with him, then made him sign his consent to exit the country. John says this man Coetzee—who had been in the background of his interrogations but till then had never exchanged a word with John—was the most chilling of all the nightmarish policemen he encountered. Coetzee went on to become South Africa's chief commissioner of police, whose job it was, until apartheid finally ended, to oversee the assassination of many opposition leaders.

John never saw his home again. By the time he was allowed to return to the country, his childhood home had been demolished. On August 6, 1969, after fifty-four days of detention, all of it in solitary confinement except for his time on the brick, he was taken directly to the airport, where he had an hour to say good-bye to his family before flying to Israel. There he lived on a kibbutz for six months rebuilding his health, before he went on to the United Kingdom, where he has lived ever since. He arrived in London as an asylum seeker, supported by student unions and charitable bodies working against apartheid. He was able to resume his studies, complete an undergraduate degree in psychology and philosophy, and secure a grant and a university place for doctoral work.

At that point, however, the burdens of everything he had been through overtook him, and he found himself unable to study.

As he recovered from this period of depression, he taught school in slums for two years, then became a psychiatric social worker and, over time, trained to become a psychotherapist.

In 1986 John helped establish a charity—the Medical Foundation for the Care of Victims of Torture—which provides rehabilitation for survivors of torture and organized violence who come to the UK from all over the world. Working there for more than twenty years, John provided direct services to clients, trained and supervised generations of staff, and produced many publications about their methods that are now used in the National Health Service in the UK.

Trauma is one key area of John's practice. He is a leading group analyst in London—his chosen therapeutic method—and a regular visitor at conferences and teaching events around the world. He holds a fellowship at University of London, where he helps run a master's program in psychotherapy, and he writes extensively.

John's abilities as a healer have clearly been strengthened by the work he has done to recover from his own history of torture, and it shows in his practice. As one of his patients at the foundation, a torture victim from Iran, said to him, "Yours is the hand of humanity that reaches out to save me from drowning in my sorrow."

And he is by no means an isolated instance. Karen Hanscom, the psychologist who founded Advocates for Survivors of Torture and Trauma in Baltimore, Maryland, says that victims of torture "always want to work with others and give back. They understand the pain that others carry. They intuitively pick up their body signals and are much more cued in to the suffering in the world. That's the step that precedes their reaching out to help."

She adds, "Torture is an experience that occurs in the context of a relationship—between torturer and victim. In order for the victim to recover, there has to be a corrective relationship experience. And sometimes a person who has been a victim of torture and is in the process of recovering is best qualified to offer such a corrective experience."

Let me conclude this piece by mentioning one of John's own heroes—Judge Albie Sachs, whom John invited to London from his native Cape Town to give an inaugural address to an international conference of psychotherapists that John helped organize. Sachs had been a longtime antiapartheid activist whose political activities while in exile had cost him an arm and the sight in one eye. (He opened a parcel bomb sent by South African security agents.) After the fall of apartheid, Sachs was appointed to the Supreme Court of the new South Africa. The new government set up a Truth and Reconciliation Commission, where perpetrators of politically directed violence were given the opportunity to acknowledge what they had done and request amnesty for their crimes. This hearing took place in the presence of their victims or the survivors of those they had killed, who also gave public testimony as to their experiences during apartheid. The commission was considered a necessary step in the transition to a democratic South Africa.

In his London speech, Sachs first recounted how he had been blown up; then, many years later, how he had worked as one of the legal architects of the Truth and Reconciliation Commission. Finally, Sachs told the story of how, while working on the country's Supreme Court, he was approached by one of the white security policemen who had tried to murder him. This man was seeking amnesty both for legal reasons and to relieve his own compelling guilt and shame. Sachs as a judge then saw this supplicant through the reconciliation process in a relationship that was first confessional and then redemptive. The story moved many to tears and provided lasting inspiration to the audience.

> *A person who has been injured always has a choice: to seek revenge, to walk away, or to extend the hand of humanity to prevent another from drowning in a sea of sorrows.*

Chapter 46

Meeting with Viktor Frankl

Everything can be taken from a man but . . . the last of the
human freedoms—to choose one's attitude in any given
set of circumstances, to choose one's own way.

—VIKTOR FRANKL, *MAN'S SEARCH FOR MEANING*

I was fortunate enough to meet Viktor Frankl in the mid-1990s, when
he was about ninety years old. At the time, he was coteaching a course
with my friend Siegfried Kasper, who is chairman of the Department of
Psychiatry and Psychotherapy at the University of Vienna. I asked Siegfried whether we might visit Frankl and, to my delight, Frankl agreed.

I had known about Viktor Frankl for years, having pored over *Man's
Search for Meaning*, his classic work that describes his experiences in the
Nazi death camps during World War II. An esteemed neurologist in
Vienna, Frankl had lost almost everything—his position, his home, his
wife, and his parents—as part of Hitler's "final solution." He himself
had been deported to a series of concentration camps, which the book
describes in painful detail. What makes the book *great*, however, is that

Frankl was able to transcend horrors by the power of his intellect, imagination, and humanity. As a doctor intrigued by the brain and the mind, Frankl not only rose above his setting but made use of it to ask a key question: In dire situations, such as a concentration camp, what can a person do to keep going? The answer, as his title suggests, is to find some meaning—something that continues to make life worth living even in the face of disaster.

For example, Frankl describes a scene in which he and a comrade are thinking of their wives. Frankl is transported by his feelings of love to a joyful and beautiful place in his mind, and feels as though he has found a profound new understanding of what love means. He also writes about the value of humor and, in a touching anecdote, describes how he tried to tutor a humorless colleague in the pleasure of a joke. Frankl used these and other insights as the basis for a form of therapy, and went on to write many more books.

As you can imagine, I was quite excited to meet someone whose life and writings I had admired for so many years. I visited Vienna in the fall of 1996, and one sunny afternoon I joined my friends Siegfried and Anita Kasper, along with Xanthi, their Lakeland terrier, to meet Frankl and his wife, Eleonore, in their summer home near the Vienna Woods.

Frankl, a short man with an upright bearing, wore flannel trousers and an open-necked cotton shirt. He looked younger than his ninety years, and had surprisingly unwrinkled skin, like someone who has never been exposed to the sun. He greeted us warmly, seemed happy to see us, and gave no impression of being a big shot. He apologized that he was losing his vision and couldn't see us too well, then led us into a study with a picture window overlooking the front lawn. The opposite wall was lined with books (most of them his). Frankl's wife, Eleonore (generally known as Elly), an attractive woman much younger than her husband, was by his side at first. During the conversation that followed, though, she remained off in the corner, as though she wished not to intrude.

Siegfried had checked with Frankl ahead of time as to whether there were any topics I should avoid, but Frankl said no, ask away. It was clear, however, that he was frail. At times during our visit, he would wince with pain; for example, at one point Xanthi barked, and his wife had to rush to give Frankl his heart medication. So my instinct was to be careful. Nevertheless, Frankl spoke candidly about the devastating loss of his family and his harrowing experiences in a death camp.

Frankl and his family had first been taken to the Terezin ghetto (also known as Theresienstadt), north of Prague. Frankl's father's health declined rapidly and he died within six months of arriving there. The following year, Frankl and his first wife, Tilly, were taken away from Terezin, leaving his mother behind. In a book about Frankl and Elly, *When Life Calls Out to Us*, Haddon Klingberg writes about the last time Frankl saw his mother.

> At the moment of their parting, Viktor asked his mother to give him her blessing. Never could he forget how she cried out from the depths of her spirit to him, "Yes! Yes! I bless you!" That was the last blessing she ever offered in Viktor's presence.

After Viktor and Tilly arrived at Auschwitz, they were separated almost immediately. Soon afterward, his mother arrived at Auschwitz as well and was murdered almost on arrival. Tilly died of exhaustion in Bergen-Belsen, about two weeks after the liberation of the camp by British troops in 1945.

As prisoners got off the train at Auschwitz, they were immediately sorted. Those sent to the right were spared to work; those sent to the left went to the gas chamber. Frankl was lucky enough to be sent to the right—perhaps because somebody coached him to put a pillow under his shirt, so his slender frame would look more robust and fit for manual labor.

Frankl was eager to talk about his work and how it differed from that of Freud, his famous Viennese colleague some fifty years his senior. The central thrust of his own work, Frankl said, was to distract a person from his problem, and encourage him to focus on other things—something he found exciting or inspiring. In contrast, he said, Freud encouraged a patient to tackle his problem directly, trying to solve it at its roots. In Frankl's view, Freud's probing moved the problem "increasingly into the central focus of the person's life, so that the person is now thinking more of his problem than of anything else, which is not necessarily in his best interests."

To illustrate his point, he shared an anecdote about the philosopher Immanuel Kant. Kant had a dear servant named Martin Lampe, who had attended to his needs for forty years. Lampe, however, began to drink excessively, and at a certain point Kant felt obliged to let him go. Upset that he had lost this man who had meant so much to him, Kant wrote himself a note, presumably as a way to comfort himself. The note, which Kant kept on his desk, said, "The name Lampe must be forgotten." Frankl smiled at the idea that the great philosopher had left himself a daily reminder of the very thing he wanted to forget. It would have been far better, in Frankl's view, for Kant to focus his attention elsewhere.

I asked Frankl whether he had ever met Freud. "Yes," he said, with enthusiasm. "On one occasion." Frankl was walking through the city when he saw an elderly man making his way to the Votive Church, in a little park now known as Sigmund Freud Park. He thought the man was muttering to himself—a psychiatric patient perhaps—but then he wondered whether it might be Freud, running his tongue over a sore in his mouth (Freud later died of oral cancer). Frankl followed the man and thought, *If he turns into the Berggasse* [the street where Freud lived], *then he is probably Freud.* In that case, Frankl would approach him.

Indeed, it was Freud. As soon as Frankl introduced himself, Freud immediately knew who he was and recited Frankl's address, which he remembered because the two had corresponded. In fact, Freud had published Frankl's first scientific paper when Frankl was still in his teens. Apparently Freud was a great correspondent and would reply to letters within a few days of receiving them. Frankl said that when you spoke to Freud, he had a special way of looking at you and listening to you. You felt your words were being carefully weighed, and that you were being taken very seriously.

I asked Frankl what had happened to him at the end of the war. He had been liberated by American troops, and after recovering his health, took a position as a doctor at a Viennese clinic, where he fell in love with a charming young nurse, Elly. Although not Jewish, Elly was no stranger to trauma. In *When Life Calls Out to Us*, Elly recalls the occupation of Vienna by Russian forces after the war. Most of her friends were raped by the troops, and one jumped out a window to her death rather than submit. Elly describes how "they even tried to rape my mother . . . they took her, in front of me, and I was standing next to three soldiers and crying. Thanks to heaven, nothing happened, but it could have very easily." Elly herself managed to avoid being raped by dressing like "a terribly dirty person" in old boots and her brother's coat, with dirt smeared on her face. Perhaps her own traumas helped Elly give Frankl the psychological support he needed, and she became his wife.

Frankl had returned to Vienna initially because he hoped to find his family, but later because that is where he wanted to live. I asked him whether he held it against the citizens of Vienna and Austria that they had been anti-Semitic and failed to protect the Jews. "No," he said emphatically. "Let us not be too self-righteous on this matter." He went on to explain that before the war, the Viennese Jewish community had been well educated and literate, whereas the Polish Jewish immigrants were less so. In fact, most of them were peasants—poorly dressed, unhygienic, and smelly, all qualities that led Austrian Jews to avoid them at times. In fact, Frankl himself had avoided sitting next to them. "I felt more like a non-Jewish Viennese than a Polish Jew," he said. His point was that nobody has a monopoly on prejudice, and everybody is capable of discrimination.

When I asked Frankl whether the Viennese could or should have done more to help their Jewish fellow citizens, he was equally firm. "It was a very dangerous time," he said. "Nobody can tell anyone else to be a hero. If you want to be a hero, that's your choice, but it's not something you can reasonably expect of anyone else."

I asked Frankl whether he forgave the Germans and Austrians for what they had done during World War II. Forgiveness, it seemed, was not a concept that Frankl related to. Instead, he valued reconciliation. Letting go of past grievances and reengaging with people seemed closer to the mark. It occurs to me that these ideas were very similar to those embraced by Nelson Mandela in dealing with the terrible injustices perpetrated under the apartheid regime. As I mentioned, under the so-called Truth and Reconciliation Committee, reconciliation was the goal; forgiveness was not a necessary part of the equation.

At one point in our conversation, I wondered whether Frankl was being too generous in his attitude. Couldn't someone have done something more? I wondered. I mentioned Elie Wiesel, another great Holocaust survivor, who has taken a far sterner view toward the actions of the German-speaking people before and during World War II. Frankl's face clouded over at this reminder. He strongly disagreed with putting a collective guilt trip on the surviving Germans and Austrians, which he regarded as unwarranted.

As Siegfried, Anita, and I piled back into Siegfried's car to return to the city, I was acutely aware that I had spent the afternoon in the company of a great man and a great healer. Even though I know that terrible psychic wounds from events like the Holocaust take decades to heal—and that old pains and grievances do return from time to time—Frankl's message of reconciliation made sense to me then, and still does. His message was helpful also to Siegfried, born to a generation of German children who were unable to ask their fathers, "Daddy, what did you do in the war?" It helped him sort out the complex relationship between Germans and Jews. In Frankl, Siegfried came to know a Jew who had suffered through the Holocaust and had survived to transmit an unusual message: "I cannot accuse someone without knowing that person's situation, if I was not there." Frankl communicated that message not only in his writings but in the gentle yet powerful way he lived his life.

> - *It is possible to survive the most terrible of ordeals and emerge from it with one's body, mind, and spirit intact.*
> - *You can find meaning even in the midst of terrible adversity.*
> - *No group of people is entirely good or evil; there are good and evil people in every group.*
> - *It is the rare person who is a hero in the sense that he or she is willing to go up against a regime of terror.*
> - *Finally, a single individual can emerge triumphant out of the rubble and live, love, speak, write, and influence millions of others.*

PART IV

FAREWELLS

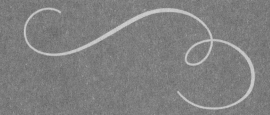

Chapter 47

A Patriarch Takes His Leave

My First Lesson in Death

It's not so bad to die.

—*THE INN OF THE SIXTH HAPPINESS*

The first dead person I ever saw was Oupa, my mother's father. Oupa had always been a strange figure to me—a successful entrepreneur, congenial but aloof, a man of few words. He had come to South Africa alone at age fourteen, at first concealed in the back of a hay wagon, which took him to a Baltic port. Then he went by ship to Cape Town. A cheap sea passage from the Baltics to Cape Town on the *Union Castle Line* made South Africa an attractive destination for Lithuanian Jews. Apparently the fares were partially subsidized by Baron de Rothschild to enable Jews to emigrate from hostile Eastern Europe to safe harbor.

At the docks in Cape Town, Oupa was met by his uncle, affectionately known to my mother and others in the family as the *Alte Gonniff* (Old Crook). How else, they reasoned, could Uncle have become so rich so fast? Had he been lucky with diamonds, which had been discovered at Kimberley shortly before he arrived in South Africa? Nobody knew; one could only speculate. But it *was* the *Alte Gonniff* who helped set Oupa up in business. He showed Oupa how to transport barrels of oil by train from Cape Town to the goldfields of Johannesburg, then pour the oil into smaller containers that could be sold to miners at a profit. Before long, Oupa had established the Pacific Oil Company—a name whose origin is mysterious, since South Africa is bounded by the Atlantic and Indian oceans, while the Pacific is thousands of miles away.

My mother would take me and my sisters to visit Oupa at his business from time to time. As I write, I recall the sweet, pungent smell of oil and see the rainbows shimmering off the oil-soaked ground. Oupa would greet us with a great smile and take us to the convenience store nearby, where he would buy us huge volumes of candy of the type that is now doled out to children in twos and threes, not in pounds. I enjoyed Oupa's candy, but we were not close. I had a sense that he knew I was one of his twelve grandchildren and could probably retrieve my name (if asked), but his attention seemed always elsewhere. His demeanor was affable but distracted—even dissociated. Perhaps a part of his mind remained behind in the old country that he had left at so young an age.

Oupa's house was his castle, where he was king. At family get-togethers, when we all sat around the large dining table, Oupa spoke while others listened. Any grandchild who dared interrupt would quickly be shushed: "Quiet! Oupa is speaking!" The rule was difficult to obey, as Oupa's stories were lengthy and repetitive. Also, some seemed to beg questioning. For example, here is why Oupa always had salt with his porridge, not sugar.

One day Dr. Welshman arrived and saw me eating my porridge with sugar. "Never do that," Dr. Welshman said. "If you want to see what that will do to your stomach, take a tin can and put porridge and sugar in it, set it in the garage for a week, then open it and see for yourself." Well, I did that and the can was full of maggots. After that, I never ate my porridge with sugar again.

Even to my five-year-old brain, something seemed wrong with the experiment. Yet I remained silent: Oupa was speaking.

Oupa had been big-boned and hardy-handsome till sickness broke him: It was a bad form of cancer. He and my grandmother moved in with us during his rapid decline. People avoided him as if cancer and death were contagious. Somehow I started visiting him in his sickbed, which would become his deathbed. He was not in pain and was always happy to see me. I think he must have been lonely.

I wish I could tell you that our conversations were fascinating. I wish I had known enough to ask how he had felt lying down in the back of the hay wagon, his parents having bribed the border guards to look the other way as a potential soldier slipped beyond reach of Czar Nicholas's recruiters. Had he been afraid? Did he worry that someone might renege on the deal? And how was it to leave his family at age fourteen and to sail halfway across the world on an ocean liner? Did someone sew gold coins into the hems of his garments? And who were his companions along the way? All those details of his youth are lost.

We do know that the *Alte Gonniff* had been Oupa's mentor of sorts, and a colorful character. Oupa had told the story of how, on one of their train rides to Johannesburg, the *Alte Gonniff* had carried packages of baked goods for friends and family. All of a sudden the police boarded the train and made straight for the *Alte Gonniff* and his luggage, sticking knitting needles into his packages to make sure they contained no illicit diamonds. (They came away empty-handed on that occasion.) None of this did I know to ask about. Instead, I accepted whatever the old man felt like talking about, which was not very much, and shared with him some ordinary details of my day. But there was a warmth to the conversation that was totally new between the two of us, and I like to think that he felt it too.

As I tell the story, I am reminded of a friend of mine who visited his father on his deathbed. The father said to him, "I'm sorry; I have nothing left to give you." Then, over the next few hours, he passed away peacefully. "He was wrong," my friend said. "Even in the last hours of his life, he gave me a great gift. He showed me how to die with dignity."

So it was with my grandfather. He made death seem not pleasant, but peaceful, painless, gentle even.

When I was eight years old, I saw the movie *The Inn of the Sixth Happiness,* starring Ingrid Bergman. To me, the most memorable scene in the movie involved a beloved old man, who was dying as those around him looked on helpless and heartbroken. He smiled weakly and comforted them. "It's not so bad to die," he said. That was a novel concept to me. Oupa's death reinforced that message.

As with many of life's profound lessons, we are destined to learn and unlearn them, and then have to learn them all over again. Years later, when I was in the dissection hall as a medical student, surrounded by cadavers, death seemed very real and terrible once more, and death by cancer worse still. I expressed my fear to one of the young surgeons teaching us anatomy. He responded, "Well, you have to die of something," and, strange as it may seem, I found comfort in that small, cold nugget of reason.

One day, several months after my grandparents' arrival, I heard a huge scream and my grandmother crying. Oupa had finally died. My mother encouraged me to visit him one last time and see him lying peacefully in his bed. The image is with me still. Visitors came, and all the rituals of mourning followed. Some commented on how kind it had been of me to keep him company when everyone else wanted to flee. To me, however, my visits had not seemed like an act of kindness. Rather, our time together was interesting and even pleasant, because, finally, Oupa became a real person to me and I to him. He knew exactly who I was, so I no longer felt like a generic grandchild. He looked forward to my visits and enjoyed them, and so did I. His final gift to me was the gift of authenticity.

The dying have unexpected gifts to offer. Be open to receiving them.

Chapter 48

Dad's Last Day

To cease upon the midnight with no pain.

—JOHN KEATS, "ODE TO A NIGHTINGALE"

When we last left my father, he was lying in a hospital bed following a heart attack, his face ashen and sweaty. Many years of physical neglect and a family tendency to heart disease had taken their toll. But he recovered from the heart attack, and lived and worked for seven more years, during which we visited to and fro. For me, those years were a bonus, but they were difficult years for Dad, who was plagued by continual anxiety and fears. It is too bad that Prozac had not yet been discovered, as he could have used it or one of its analogues.

If Dad could have scripted his own death, he could hardly have done better (though at age sixty-seven, it was a bit early). He died on his birthday. It was a quick death—almost as easy as death can be. The day itself was joyful. He always used to joke that you knew your son had made it in the United States when he called and didn't reverse the charges. Long-distance calls were expensive back then, but I remember on that day actually deciding that it was time to call with my own money, a fact he proudly related to his secretary when he got to work.

The whole day was one of celebration, as friends dropped by his office. He capped it off in a restaurant with my mother, sister, and brother-in-law, where he ate his favorite dinner—fried steak and eggs (off-limits of course, for a cardiac patient). Shortly afterward he felt ill and my brother-in-law rushed him to the hospital. At some point in the journey, Dad reached over, yanked the handbrake—as though he thought he were driving and had to stop the car—groaned, and was gone.

One of his friends put it best when he said, "I think Charlie would have preferred it this way. He would not have enjoyed languishing for years and, frankly, he would have been a rotten patient." I have now seen several of my friends' parents live into their eighties and nineties, gradually declining in body and mind. In some cases, they no longer recognize their children or know where they are. Many are perpetually confused and frightened. People sometimes pay a heavy price for those extra years.

I am left wondering whether it is better to fade gradually into the sunset and die in one's late eighties or to go suddenly at the height of one's mental powers in the mid-sixties. It is a question best left to the gods. In Dad's case, they decided to take him quickly, which, in retrospect, seems kind.

I grieved for Dad a long while, not only for the loss but also for the sorrows of his life, for which there seemed to be no steady remedy.

Sometimes a rapid exit is kindest.

Chapter 49

The Death of Galadriel

Farewell to Middle-earth at last.
I see the Star above my mast!

—J. R. R. TOLKIEN

My sister-in-law, whom I will call Galadriel, was a striking young woman—tall and willowy, with a pale, clear complexion and flowing brown hair. She wore long, flower-patterned dresses in the fashion of the folksingers of the seventies and often had an otherworldly expression. She gave the impression of someone with access to a realm beyond the humdrum drudgery of daily life.

For a career, she had decided to follow her talent and her passion for ancient music, playing both the lute and flute as her chosen instruments. For entertainment she read fantasy stories, her favorite being Tolkien's *Lord of the Rings*, which she consumed from cover to cover (all twelve hundred pages) at least twelve times. It is fair to say that she inhabited Tolkien's world for many of her waking hours. I never discussed with her which character she most identified with, but the one she most resembled is Galadriel, "the mightiest and fairest of all the Elves that remained in Middle Earth."

Having learned all she could from her music teacher in South Africa, Galadriel moved to Holland in 1979 to work with a master there. She also went to Germany to purchase a very special new lute, with which she started back to Holland by train. As the train crossed the border, however, she was accosted by a German train official, who interrogated her in German about the lute. She understood no German and was unable to answer his questions. He then took her into another compartment and left her there alone. Afterward, he explained that he had gone to find an English translator, but it was never clear why more interviewing would require that she be left alone. She must have been terrified, perhaps remembering scenes of interrogation from movies about World War II. Why else would a young woman just blooming into an international career in a field that she loved do what she did?—which was jump out the window of a rapidly moving train. And that was the end of Galadriel.

Years later, while traveling across Germany by train with Josh, I had an encounter with a German train conductor that reminded me of this incident. Josh had been accosted by the conductor and, not understanding what the problem was, Josh called me to assist him. On inspecting our Eurail passes, the conductor began to scream at me in high-speed German. In the United States, people would be ashamed to speak to their dogs in such a tone. I was eventually able to decipher that Josh and I had failed to have our Eurail passes stamped at the point of embarkation, which one is required to do. Well, I thought, this must happen all the time, so there must be some established procedure. But the conductor had no interest in a remedy. He continued to berate and insult me.

The conductor and I were both standing in the coach and, cornered by this rottweiler, I remembered Galadriel, and my heart went out to her all over again. Somehow this rabid man helped me see her final act of desperation—ghastly as it was—as less strange, more understand-able. I looked at him and said, "I don't know what you expect me to do, but I'm not jumping out the window." Of course, even had he under-stood a word of English, the statement would have made no sense to him.

The most astonishing aspect of the scene was that the bystanders, well-dressed men and women, all sat by and allowed this diatribe to continue. Didn't someone know English? I wondered. Couldn't anyone help? I turned to them and said, "Is this how you treat visitors to your country? After your history, aren't you ashamed to let someone talk to a guest in this way?" They started to squirm in their seats and suddenly everyone began to help. They settled down, and one man stepped in as interpreter. He explained the problem to me and told me that I needed to pay several hundred marks to correct my mistake, which of course I did. The Sturm und Drang was resolved simply by paying a fine. Why didn't the conductor say so in the first place? I wondered. But I knew the answer: He didn't want a resolution; he wanted a fight—and to show me who was boss.

AS JOSH AND I returned to our seats, the train conductor was still fuming. Apparently he felt that his authority had been undermined. He requested my U.S. passport and saw "Rosenthal" written on it. I can't imagine what he thought of that, but later, when he came along with the cart, he declined to sell me and Josh pastries. Perhaps I was merely unlucky to come up against a pathologically aggressive conductor, just as perhaps my sister-in-law had been. Perhaps it could have happened anywhere. But the incident gave me a visceral feeling for history, for how lucky I was to be a Jew on a German train in 1990, not 1940. And how lucky it is for so many people that the rules have changed dramati-cally and fundamentally since those terrible times.

Another thing the incident did for me was to fill me with pro-found compassion for Galadriel—a delicate person, alone, with perhaps a tenuous grip on reality. I now understand better how an encounter with a brutal official could have pushed her over the edge and to her death.

> *Stand up to bullies whenever you safely can, and recruit others in that venture whenever possible.*

Chapter 50

Appointment in Samarra

Everybody has got to die, but I always believed an exception
would be made in my case.

—WILLIAM SAROYAN

This thou perceiv'st, which makes thy love more strong,
To love that well which thou must leave ere long.

—SHAKESPEARE, SONNET 73

The quote by short-story writer William Saroyan shown above encapsulates one of the mysteries of death: We know that death is inevitable (including our own), but it is nonetheless unimaginable. We have
known the world only from our own viewpoint, a world with ourselves
at its center. What would a world without us—without me!—be like?
The imagination falters when we think of that moment when our own
consciousness ceases. No wonder death is so scary!

The title of this chapter comes from a story that has been told in
different forms and languages, but most famously perhaps by Somerset
Maugham. Here is his version, as told by Death:

There was a merchant in Baghdad who sent his servant to market to buy provisions and in a little while the servant came back, white and trembling, and said, "Master, just now when I was in the marketplace I was jostled by a woman in the crowd and when I turned I saw it was Death that jostled me. She looked at me and made a threatening gesture. Now, lend me your horse, and I will ride away from this city and avoid my fate. I will go to Samarra and there Death will not find me." The merchant lent him his horse, and the servant mounted it, and he dug his spurs in its flanks and as fast as the horse could gallop, he went. Then the merchant went down to the marketplace and he saw me standing in the crowd and he came to me and said, "Why did you make a threatening gesture to my servant when you saw him this morning?" "That was not a threatening gesture," I said, "It was only a start of surprise. I was astonished to see him in Baghdad, for I had an appointment with him tonight in Samarra."

The message of Maugham's story—and the reality of death—can be summed up by the commonly used expression, "You can run, but you can't hide."

As a young man, stabbed and bleeding en route to the emergency room, I realized I could be dying and thought, *That would be okay,* which was comforting. Perhaps I was merely responding to the endorphins flooding my body, for later, when I was married with a child, I certainly wanted to stay alive with every fiber of my being. So it seems as though our feelings about dying change according to our time of life, our circumstances, and our brain chemistry. At least, that's how it has been for me, and for many I have seen in various stages of dying.

When I have been powerfully focused on a goal, like anticipating Josh's wedding, visiting my aging mother in South Africa, or completing a writing or research project, I have sometimes thought, *Not now— this would not be a good time to die.* Then invariably I smile at myself. Do I really think death will wait till I decide that the time is right to die? And, indeed, is there *ever* a good time to die? I smile too at Emily Dickinson's immortal words: "Because I could not stop for Death, He kindly stopped for me." With beautiful irony, she seems to be saying, "How nice of Death to realize how busy I was and pick me up personally instead of waiting for me to be ready."

That whole notion of a time for dying brings to mind an old brainteaser in which a mathematics professor says to his class, "You will get a math test on one day next week, but only if the day in question is a surprise." The students reason that it cannot be Friday because if Thursday has passed, there will be only one day left in the week, so a Friday test would be no surprise. By the same logic, the students go on to exclude Thursday (if by the end of Wednesday there had been no test . . .) and all the other days. The following Wednesday, the professor walks into class and hands out the test—which is, indeed, a surprise. This logic problem has been called the Unexpected Hanging Paradox because one popular variation of the problem involves a prisoner who faces hanging, not a student about to take an exam. Logicians do not agree on a definitive solution to the problem. What fascinates me about the paradox, however, more than whatever logical flaws it presumably contains, is that it reminds me of the way so many of us think about death (if we think about it at all). We know it's going to happen, but we find reasons for why it shouldn't happen today, or tomorrow, or any day next week, for that matter. Yet, presto! It happens—and sure enough, we are surprised.

Death can surprise not only by when it occurs but also by how— which can be freakishly unpredictable. On first reading that the Greek dramatist Aeschylus reportedly died when struck by a falling tortoise, dropped from the beak of an eagle, it occurred to me that a person could die suddenly and unexpectedly from pretty much anything coming (in this case literally) out of the blue. Though the story is probably apocryphal, its essence remains true to my experience. Eagles *do* drop tortoises, just as gulls drop oysters, to get at the meat by smashing the shell. Someone *might* easily be walking underneath, and the blow could certainly be fatal. Closer to home, I read about a ninety-year-old woman who was crushed by a falling tree while she slept. Each day, perhaps this woman might have gone about her activities with every reasonable expectation of an ordinary death. Yet, when the time came, her violent demise was probably so quick she didn't even have time to be surprised.

S. Srirangam Shreeram (better known to us all as Shree), a psychiatrist of South Indian origin, was a friend and colleague who worked in my medical research organization. He was a tall, handsome man, quiet, dignified, and intellectually gifted. Everyone loved and respected him. One day he came into work, complaining of back pain. The next day he went to the emergency room after his back muscles went into unbearably painful spasms. He was admitted to the hospital and, though he received superb care, we never saw him again. He made the diagnosis himself—rabies—and asked that he be bound to the bed railings to stop him from infecting anyone else.

Some months before, Shree had visited his family in India, where, during his morning jog, he was scratched by a stray dog. We all know rabies can be transmitted by a dog bite, but a dog scratch? Who ever heard of that? After the jog, Shree returned home, washed and disinfected the wound, and thought no more about it.

Rabies vaccine, given even after a person is infected, is almost 100 percent effective at preventing the disease by causing the body to produce antibodies to the virus. If you are infected and do *not* get the vaccine, however, the viruses from the animal's saliva make their way into the peripheral nerve endings at the wound site. From there they travel slowly up the nerves toward the central nervous system, where they so irritate the brain and spinal cord that even the slightest stimulus can trigger terrible spasms. The rabid dog that infected Shree must have licked its paw, leaving infected saliva on its claws and thus in the scratch.

Only a few people contract rabies in the United States each year;

almost all of them die. You are about two hundred times more likely to be hit by lightning. Yet this awful disease killed someone I knew well. Recognizing the unpredictability of fate, the ancient Greeks used to say, "Count no man happy until he is dead."

While it is not sensible to walk about fearing a freakishly unlikely death, in many situations, death is predictable—for example, in an old person dying of cancer. Even then, however, denial of death is common, which has consequences for society as a whole. For example, a high proportion of the U.S. Medicare budget goes toward end-of-life care: a third of all Medicare costs provide care for the last year of life, a third of which covers the final month.

For the individual, such denial of death can be costly, preventing people from taking out life insurance or making proper estate plans. A small-town lawyer once told me about a couple, Ermil and Ruby, who asked him to draft their wills. But the couple delayed and delayed when it came to signing the documents. Whenever he saw them in the supermarket or at the bank, he would say, "You should stop by and sign those wills sometime." One day the lawyer read in the local newspaper that Ruby had died; later that same day Ermil called. The lawyer offered condolences. Ermil thanked him and said, "By the way, would it be okay for me to stop by and sign our wills later today?"

At the opposite extreme are those who deliberately and regularly remind themselves of their own mortality. It is a common element in many religions. Metaphysical poet John Donne is said to have slept in his own coffin and worn his own shroud—extreme behavior even for the time, but understandable from the man who wrote "Death be not proud." Celebrated actress Sarah Bernhardt frequently slept in a coffin, claiming that it helped her better understand her tragic roles.

One of the most unusual and elaborate approaches in the annals of courtship was surely that of seventeenth-century poet Andrew Marvell, who attempted to persuade his coy mistress to set aside her chastity by reminding her that:

The grave's a fine and private place,
But none, I think, do there embrace.

We have no record as to whether his approach succeeded, but you have to give him points for trying, and the resulting poem is an acknowledged masterpiece.

IN MODERN TIMES, people seldom to never commission a portrait of themselves staring at a skull, but many still remember the value of being mindful of death throughout life. Steve Jobs, the late founder of Apple, told a group of graduating Stanford students that his daily awareness of his own mortality shaped his life decisions. For years he would ask himself each day whether, if that day were his last, he would spend it as planned. If the answer were no too many days in a row, he would reevaluate his goals.

Shakespeare wrote often and poignantly about the ravages of time and argued that we should use this awareness to heighten and intensify feelings of love—"to love that well which thou must leave ere long."

> *Awareness of your own mortality can sharpen your feelings and sense of purpose. Use that awareness to make sure your actions reflect what is most important in your life.*
>
> *Such awareness can also strengthen the bonds between you and your loved ones.*

Chapter 51

Life After Death

Remember me when I am gone away
Gone far away into the silent land.
—CHRISTINA ROSSETTI

A friend of mine spent a pleasant afternoon sitting with his mother in the shade of a large tree. His mother, who was in the final stages of a terminal disease, turned to him and said, "I'll miss you when I'm gone." They smiled at each other, understanding both what she meant and the humor of the statement.

The question of what happens after we die is a great mystery that perfuses our lives. Once the body has died, is there an aspect of the "self" that survives—and, if so, what happens to it? I recently read an interview with Stephen Hawking, arguably one of the world's greatest living scientists, in which he compared people to computers in that our consciousness results from neurons firing. According to his reasoning, when we die, we cease to be conscious, much as a broken computer stops processing information. Hawking sees the hereafter as a fairy tale that people use to comfort themselves; there is no hereafter, he says, for broken computers.

On the other end of the spectrum are those who believe in the soul and a divine immortal energy of some sort, and who have detailed descriptions of what happens to the soul after death. Many expect divine rewards or punishments for good and evil deeds performed in life. Such ideas led philosopher Blaise Pascal, ever the statistician, to provide a logical argument for believing in God: If your faith is mistaken, you've lost nothing. But if God does exist and rewards believers, then you will be sitting pretty when the time comes.

Wherever you are on that spectrum is no business of mine. I just wanted to acknowledge these competing theories about life after death in order to set them clearly aside and return to my friend's mother, who was telling him not only that she loved him but also that she wanted him to remember that after she was gone. Christina Rossetti (quoted above) also wants to be remembered after her death—if only for a while. So it is that people express a certain kind of "life after death"— they want you to know how they would feel if they were alive, even after they no longer are.

I have conducted a thought experiment on myself and some friends as follows: Imagine that there is a nuclear holocaust in which everyone in the world dies. Then, in a second scenario, imagine that only you die (in some quick and painless way). Which scenario feels worse to contemplate?

Most people say that the holocaust is much worse—even those who don't believe in life after death. I find that interesting, because once you're dead, what difference does it make to you whether others are alive or not? Yet for most people it does. We are concerned about life after death—the life of others after our own death.

We see this concern for life after death in the common desire to leave a legacy. A friend of mine, a psychologist in his eighties, who, when I last saw him, was having more fun than most people half his age, claims to be an exception to this rule. "I have no interest in leaving a legacy," he told me. "All I care about is enjoying my life." It sounded good, but as I saw all the things he was still doing for other people and to make the world a better place, there seemed to be an element of bravado in his claim. My guess is that many people, if not most, care about leaving a legacy. Why else would anybody do research, write a book, design a building, found a charity, enact legislation, or do anything else that consumes many days of their life rather than just have a good time? You could argue that many of these people will live to see the fruits of their labor, but in most cases, they also want their accomplishments to survive their time on earth. They want to feel that their own lives have made a difference, a difference that will continue even after they die.

When she reached her eighties, my mother embarked on a new project. She decided she would crochet an afghan for each of her children, grandchildren, nieces, and nephews, each in the recipient's favorite colors. On one of my trips home, Mom casually asked me whether I would like her to crochet an afghan for me. When I readily accepted, she said, "Let's go to the wool shop and choose the colors together."

I have the afghan still, spread out in a place of honor. So do many others in the family. The message of the blankets was clear: Mom wanted to keep us warm long after she was gone. When we saw their bright colors, she wanted us to be cheerful—and perhaps even to remember her own vividness and vibrancy. She wanted us to know that each of us mattered to her—as did our individual tastes in color.

The puzzle of altruism has long been debated among scholars of evolution. If the genes that drive our behavior are so selfish, they wonder, why do we see examples of altruism all around—in this case altruism that drives one to care about the well-being of others even after one's own death? The latest theory, expounded most famously by sociobiologist E. O. Wilson, is that as different groups of organisms compete with one another, those groups that take care of their members will have an advantage in the battle for survival. Or perhaps you would prefer to see caretaking as an aspect of love. Both could be true.

The topic of this chapter is especially timely, because in the decades ahead, as the world's population grows, as our resources shrink, and as the ecology of the planet becomes more and more precarious, Earth is likely to become an increasingly inhospitable place. Competition among groups is likely to be fierce. But at the same time, collaboration among the world's people and nations will be essential to human survival, and the sooner we start, the better. Now, more than ever, is the time to care about life after death, and invest in it.

> *If we care about the future of our loved ones and of all humanity, it is important to consider life after death—their life and our death.*

Chapter 52

It's Never Too Late to Say "I Love You"

I like not only to be loved, but also to be told that
I am loved; the realm of silence is large enough
beyond the grave.

—GEORGE ELIOT

When my mother approached her mid-eighties, her heart began to fail. Good medical care kept her going, but medications can do only so much. I visited twice a year and with each visit saw changes—she'd lost weight; her step had slowed. She was slipping away.

My mother always had difficulty expressing emotions, or so she said.

"I'm just not emotional," she would declare. "Or verbal. Your father is the verbal one."

Often, when we would talk by phone over the ten thousand miles that separate the United States from South Africa, she would run out of things to say about herself. But she had an unusual quality. She would actually remember what I had said in a previous conversation, and she'd follow up when next we talked. "How are the ants?" she'd ask. Or "Is the smell of paint gone yet?" She'd be asking these questions long after I had forgotten about the exterminator's visit or that we'd had a room repainted.

As she approached the end of her life, her mind became less laser-sharp than it had been, but she was still able to distill things to their essence. We had discussed some years before that when she died, it was unlikely that I would be there with her, given the ten thousand miles. "I know," she said. "But there is always the telephone."

A week or so before she died, I remembered her saying that. I was in Vancouver for a professional meeting, and during a walk in the majestic Stanley Park, I found a public phone and called her.

"How are you, Mom?" I asked.

"I'm happy," she said. "I'm happy." It sounded true, although I also wondered whether, even as she lay dying, she sought to comfort me.

When she died, one of my sisters and I flew back to Johannesburg, where Mom had lived with my other sister. After the funeral, the prayers, and the visitors, we went looking for her will. She had little by way of money or possessions, but we knew that this was an important step. We wanted to hold on to any last link with her.

We found the will—a simple document, dividing everything three ways. No surprises there. The surprise came in the form of the following undated letter, enclosed with the will, and excerpted here:

Dear Children:

I feel that during my lifetime I haven't told you sufficiently often how much I love you. You have been three shining lights throughout my life. . . .

You have been a mother's pride and joy!!

I wish you all a long and healthy life, and have as much pleasure and happiness from your children as I have had from mine.

Esta

Our grief swept over us like a tidal wave and we cried our eyes out, but they were good tears, necessary tears. My brother-in-law shut the doors to give us privacy, and we kept crying until we were worn-out.

My mother's letter sits in a drawer beside my desk, and I read it from time to time. Her words continue to inspire and encourage me to try to do my best, and to be as kind as I can, both to others and to myself.

It is never too late to say "I love you."

ACKNOWLEDGMENTS

I am grateful to many people who helped bring this book to fruition. I owe thanks to two superb editors: Mitch Horowitz, editor in chief at Tarcher/Penguin, who believed in this project and helped shape it; and Elise Hancock, who helped in countless ways to improve my earlier drafts. Thanks also to those who read through earlier versions and provided invaluable feedback, particularly Leora Rosen and Wendy Lachman.

Special thanks to the following people for their key contributions: my classmate Lucille Berro and her mother, Sylvia Berro, for sharing Sylvia's amazing story of survival; Tom Wehr for helping me reconstruct events that occurred at the National Institute of Mental Health; Julian Karpoff for his insights and expertise; Bobby Roth and Mario Orsatti for their help with the chapter on the value of meditation for people dealing with extreme hardship; John Schlapobersky for generously sharing the details of his own struggle in apartheid South Africa, his expertise on the effects of trauma, and many facts about our family's history; Siegfried and Anita Kasper for introducing me to Viktor Frankl; Siegfried Kasper and Harald Mori (former assistant to Viktor Frankl) for their help in making sure I got my facts straight about the terrible details of the war years and Frankl's contributions after the war; and

Lois Lee and the Children of the Night program for helping me understand the problems of young street workers in Los Angeles.

Thanks are also due to many, many people for offering their own stories and recollections, and providing expert commentary and insights. I have deliberately withheld the identities of some of the people in this book in order to safeguard their privacy; please accept my gratitude anonymously. Happily, I am able to name the following individuals for helping in so many ways: Derek Barnett, Ora Baumgarten, Larry Blossom, Danny Cohen, Christine Courtois, Ray Dalio, Eric Finzi, Rod Freedman, Rick Friedman, Shebna Garcon, Chris Germer, Jennifer and Cedric Ginsberg, Karen Hanscom, Jay Hoofnagle, Kay Redfield Jamison, Stacy King, Desmond Lachman, Peter Lachman, Karen Lawrence, Lois Lee, Susan and Wilfred Lieberthal, Michael Liebowitz, Ian Livingstone, David Lynch, Dan McQuaid, Hilda Ochoa-Brillembourg, Pamela Peeke, James Pennebaker, Kenneth and Lydia Polonsky, Marian and Peter Prinsley, Rusty Rostowsky, Simon Shapiro, Cadi Simon, Catherine Tuggle, Colin Vaines, and Barry Zito.

Finally, my love and thanks to Leora and Joshua, for being such an integral part of my life, and for all your kindness and support.

APPENDIX

JAMES W. PENNEBAKER'S WRITING EXERCISE

1. For the best results, take the exercise seriously and make a commitment to follow through on all phases of the exercise. The goal of the exercise is to reveal your deepest secrets to yourself in an honest way. To do this, you need to "get into" your writing as deeply as possible.

2. Even though the total writing-time commitment is less than ninety minutes, it is important to take this time commitment seriously. Be sure to schedule four twenty-minute undisturbed blocks of time into your schedule on four consecutive days.

3. If at all possible, find a quiet place that is away from the ordinary hurly-burly of your life, away from telephones and other sources of distraction. The idea is to immerse yourself in your writing for these few short blocks of time. The best results are obtained when you find a special place where you can focus exclusively on your writing.

4. The only rule of the writing exercise is to write continuously for the entire twenty minutes. If you run out of things to say, just repeat what you have already written. In your writing, don't worry about grammar, spelling, or sentence structure. Just write.

5. Sometimes people feel a little sad or depressed after writing. If this happens, it is completely normal. Most people say that these feelings go away in an hour or so.

6. Be sure that your writing is completely anonymous and confidential. If you have any concern that someone else will find your written material, it may constrain what you say and how you say it, which may make the exercise less effective.

7. What you should write about over the four days is the most traumatic, upsetting experience in your entire life. In your writing, you should really let go and explore your very deepest emotions and thoughts. You can write about the same experience on all four days or about different experiences each day. In addition to a traumatic experience, you can also write about major conflicts or problems that you have experienced or are experiencing now. Whatever you choose to write, however, it is critical that you really delve into your deepest emotions and thoughts. Ideally, you should also write about significant experiences that you have not discussed in great detail with others. Remember that you have four days to write. You can tie your traumatic experience to other parts of your life: how it is related to your childhood, your parents, the people you love, who you are, or who you want to be. Again, in your writing, examine your deepest emotions and thoughts.

8. When you finish the writing exercise, you can keep the written materials or throw them away. Remember, the key to this strategy is the exercise itself and not the quality of the finished product.

Source: James Pennebaker. *Opening Up*, Guilford Press, 1997

INDEX

ABOUT THE AUTHOR

Norman E. Rosenthal is the world-renowned psychiatrist, researcher, and author, who first described seasonal affective disorder (SAD) and pioneered the use of light therapy as a treatment during his twenty years at the National Institute of Mental Health. A highly cited researcher and best-selling author, he has written over 200 scholarly articles, and authored or coauthored eight popular books. These include *Winter Blues*, the *New York Times* best seller *Transcendence*, and the *The Gift of Adversity*. He has practiced psychiatry for over three decades, coached, and conducted numerous clinical trials of medications and alternative treatments, such as Transcendental Meditation, for psychiatric disorders. He and his work have been featured on *Good Morning America*, *The Today Show*, NPR, and other national media.

Also by Norman E. Rosenthal, M.D.

TRANSCENDENCE

Healing and Transformation Through Transcendental Meditation

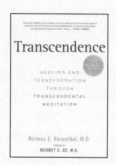